Infections in Children

A Sourcebook for Educators and Child Care Providers

Second Edition

Infections in Children

A Sourcebook for Educators and Child Care Providers

Second Edition

Richard D. Andersen, MD
Children's Hospital of St. Paul
St. Paul, Minnesota

James A. Blackman, MD, MPH
Kluge Children's Rehabilitation Center
University of Virginia
Charlottesville, Virginia

James F. Bale, Jr., MD
Department of Pediatrics & Neurology
The University of Iowa
Iowa City, Iowa

Jody R. Murph, MD
Department of Pediatrics
The University of Iowa
Iowa City, Iowa

AN ASPEN PUBLICATION®
Aspen Publishers, Inc.
Gaithersburg, Maryland
1994

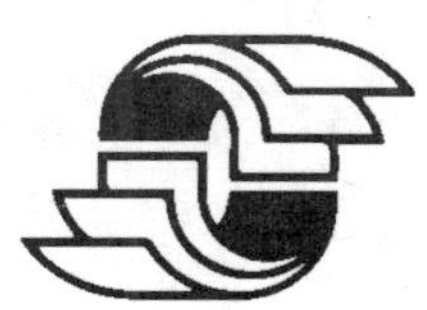

Library of Congress Cataloging-in-Publication Data

Infections in Children/Richard D. Andersen . . . [et al.]. -2nd ed.
p. cm.
Includes bibliographical references and index.
ISBN 0-8342-0387-1
1. Infection in children. 2. Communicable diseases in children.
I. Andersen, Richard D.
RJ401.I54 1994
618.92'9--dc20
93-30760
CIP

Editorial Services: Barbara Priest
Amy Martin

The authors have made every effort to ensure the accuracy of the information herein, particularly with regard to drug selection and dose. However, appropriate information sources should be consulted, especially for new or unfamiliar drugs or procedures. It is the responsibility of every practitioner to evaluate the appropriateness of a particular opinion in the context of actual clinical situations and with due consideration to new developments Authors, editors, and the publisher cannot be held responsible for any typographical or other errors found in this book.

Library of Congress Catalog Card Number: 93-30760
ISBN: 0-8342-0387-1

Printed in the United States of America

1 2 3 4 5

This book is dedicated to our children Katie, Sara, Michael, Jeremy, David, Meghan, Zachary, Jeffrey, Margaret, Elizabeth, Carl, and Kathryn.

Table of Contents

Preface

In reviewing the medical landscape since the first edition of this book, we find rapid changes in the world of infectious diseases of children. The discouraging expansion of acquired immunodeficiency syndrome in the pediatric population has been accompanied by new hope for life-prolonging treatment strategies and massive research efforts on human immunodeficiency virus. The promise of the 1980s of a new vaccine to reduce dramatically childhood meningitis is a promise fulfilled in the 1990s. As we witness a potential proliferation of other new and safe vaccines, we must also note the declining will of both parents and health care providers to immunize our nation's children. While our possibilities for disease eradication expand, old issues such as measles and tuberculosis resurface and remind us of the continuing vulnerabilities of today's children.

Child care providers, educators, and parents who struggle with the increasingly complex issues of childhood infection need updated information. The authors have appreciated comments from the readers of the first edition and hope that this volume meets their needs and expectations.

HOW TO USE THIS BOOK

The authors recognize that readers in different settings have used this book for different purposes. This edition has been organized so that the first section (Chapters 1–6) might serve as a primer on infections and could be read as a whole, for example, by new employees in a school or child-care setting. The remainder of the book might be used as a reference when specific infectious disease problems arise.

Acknowledgments

The authors would like to thank Pat Moore and Cindy Thorson, who assisted in the preparation of this manuscript.

Part I

General Considerations for Group Settings

Chapter 1

Introduction: Infectious Disease in Children

From birth to adolescence, children live in a world in which viruses, bacteria, and other microorganisms greatly outnumber human beings. Most of these "germs" live in harmony with humans, but others (termed pathogens) can cause disease. The "germ theory" of infectious diseases is a relatively new concept. Until the last few centuries, most infectious diseases were believed to be caused by forces of nature, actions of individuals, or divine intervention. In the 17th century, scientists discovered microbes and began investigating the role they play in causing human disease. This discovery revolutionized concepts of infection and set the stage for developments such as immunization and drug therapy. The search for microbes continues today, but with a dramatic reduction in the time it takes to track down a causative agent. Legionnaires' disease and acquired immunodeficiency syndrome are two examples of how intensive investigative efforts have yielded virtually instantaneous (in historical terms) discovery of the cause.

FACTORS THAT DETERMINE THE LIKELIHOOD OF INFECTION

Several factors help determine whether an encounter between host and microbe will result in disease. One is the intrinsic capacity of an organism to cause disease (virulence). A good example of a highly virulent agent is the rabies virus. The mere presence of this organism in the nonimmune human host is uniformly fatal. A second important determinant is the number or "dose" of microorganisms. For instance, diarrhea-causing salmonella bacteria, if ingested in small numbers, can be destroyed by stomach acid. If the number of organisms exceeds that which the stomach acid can effectively destroy, however, diarrheal illness results. A third factor in determining whether a microbe–host encounter will result in disease is the status of the individual child. This includes not only specific immunity (eg, from previous exposure to chickenpox) but also general factors such as nutritional status, underlying disease, and drug therapy. The skin, mucous membranes, and gastrointestinal tract are covered (colonized) with millions of microorganisms, primarily bacteria, that constitute what is called the normal flora. These organisms cause infection only when immune responses are suppressed or when the usual defense barriers are broken down (eg, through surgery).

A CHILD'S IMMUNE SYSTEM

Our understanding of microbes and the role they play in human health evolved over many decades. In contrast, discoveries about the complexities of the immune system (immunology) have been more explosive and recent. Moreover, the number of persons who are immunosuppressed (also termed immunocompromised) is increasing with the continuing expansion and success of cancer chemotherapy and other immunosuppressive drugs and because of acquired immunodeficiency syndrome.

Organs and Cells of the Immune System

The immune system, one of the body's many organ systems, is the group of organs and cells primarily responsible for defending the body against infection. Various body components serve as immune organs: The bone marrow in certain parts of the body behaves as a kind of factory for producing immune cells; the spleen, lymph nodes, and, to some extent, the liver serve as filters to remove microorganisms; and the thymus produces certain white blood cells. All these organs are especially rich in white blood cells, the cells primarily responsible for host defense. The blood stream makes it possible for these white cells to move to any part of the body.

During the 19th century, a debate raged over how the body destroys invaders. One side maintained that immune cells actually engulf microorganisms (phagocytosis); the other side argued that the actual destroyers are not the immune cells themselves but the substances they produce (what we now call antibodies).

It is now clear that both sides were correct. Humans have two kinds of immunity—cellular and humoral—and the network of interactions among immune cells is extraordinarily complex. The actual engulfment of microorganisms (phagocytosis) is carried out primarily by two kinds of white blood cells: the neutrophils and the macrophages. The macrophages also interact with yet another type of white blood cell; the lymphocytes. There are two categories of lymphocytes: T cells and B cells. Certain T cells kill virus-infected target cells. Other T cells (called helper cells) help other immune cells carry out their functions. B cells, in contrast, secrete antibodies in plasma. These antibodies, also known as gamma globulins, are of five types: immunoglobulin M (IgM), IgG, IgA, IgE, and IgD. Some antibodies (the IgM type) make a short-term response to acute infection. Other antibodies (IgG) are long term and may circulate for a lifetime. These are the antibodies that prevent someone who had measles at age 5 from contracting it again at age 55. Over the years, as various organisms are encountered and combatted, the body accumulates a repertoire of antibodies (the immune memory). This helps explain why children are more susceptible than adults to common infections.

Stages of Immune System Development

The child's immune system undergoes roughly three stages of development: the newborn period, the infant-toddler period, and the school-age period. Each group has its own special vulnerabilities to disease.

Newborns (infants younger than 1 month) are especially vulnerable to infection. There are many organisms against which the newborn's relatively underdeveloped immune system does not provide adequate protection. An example is herpes simplex virus, which can cause devastating infection. The immune system of the newborn is particularly underdeveloped in its capacity for producing IgA, the primary immune globulin of secretions. (Breast milk is rich in IgA and thus may help protect the gastrointestinal tract from certain microorganisms, a benefit that is particularly evident in countries where diarrhea-causing microorganisms are widespread.)

Newborns are not equally vulnerable to all microorganisms, however. One reason is that certain activities of the immune system (eg, some T-lymphocyte functions) appear to be relatively well developed at birth. In addition, some of the mother's immune factors are transmitted to the fetus via the placenta. For example, if the mother has antibodies to measles, her child is also protected during pregnancy and for months after delivery. The antibodies accumulated over a lifetime by the mother thus serve as a protective umbrella for the infant, with individual antibodies lasting anywhere from a few months to a year, depending on the level and type. Once these antibodies have disappeared, however, the child is immunologically naked until vaccines or natural diseases re-create specific antibodies. This is one reason why children contract many more community illnesses in the period from 6 to 12 months of age than they do during the first 6 months of life.

By the end of the first year of life, most or all of the immunities received from the mother have vanished, and children typically have a multitude of infectious encounters, especially in the respiratory and gastrointestinal tracts. Between the ages of 6 months and 2 years, children have a new range of vulnerabilities. There is an increased prevalence of certain bacterial infections. For example, in the 1980s before immunization, approximately 1 child in every 400 experienced meningitis caused by the bacterium *Hemophilus influenzae* (see Chapter 9), a condition that seldom occurs in other age groups. Such vulnerabilities may reflect not only the loss of maternal antibodies but also an inability to generate a satisfactory immune response to certain organisms.

By the time a child enters kindergarten, the immune system is relatively mature. Between the ages of 3 and 6 years the immune response is particularly exuberant, as manifested by enlarged tonsils and "swollen glands" in the neck. (Before physicians recognized that this lymphoid activity is normal and temporary, tonsillectomy was a routine operation for children in this age group.)

MICROORGANISMS

Childhood diseases can be caused by viruses, bacteria, and other microorganisms. Distinguishing between viral and bacterial organisms is often the key issue in diagnosing and treating disease, largely because bacteria respond to antibiotic treatment and viruses do not.

Microbiologists (scientists engaged in the study of microbes) classify disease-causing microorganisms into categories, which are described here in order of their structural complexity, from smallest to largest.

Viruses

In a strict sense, viruses are not microorganisms because they are only fragments of living forms that reside in other cells and use cell machinery to reproduce themselves. Viruses are made up of genetic material (DNA or RNA) and a protective covering. Virtually all viruses have specific preferences (tropisms) for the type of cells they inhabit. Some, such as herpes simplex virus and varicella-zoster (chickenpox, shingles) virus, can exist in a hidden (latent) state within the body for decades. Most viral illnesses are diagnosed by clinical examination or not at all. This is because viruses are difficult to culture: They are too small to be seen under standard microscopes and they require particular host cells that can be maintained only in special diagnostic virology laboratories.

Chlamydia, Mycoplasma, and *Rickettsia* Organisms

These three types of organisms have some features of viruses and some features of bacteria. Chlamydial disease is a leading sexually transmitted disease that can result in conjunctivitis and pneumonia in newborns. Mycoplasma infections are predominantly respiratory (see Chapter 10), whereas rickettsial diseases [which include Rocky Mountain spotted fever (see Chapter 13)] can involve the skin and many other organs. A limited number of antibiotics are useful in treating infections with these three groups of microorganisms.

Bacteria

Bacteria are abundant in nature. The moment humans emerge from the virtually sterile environment of the womb, they are colonized with millions of bacteria. Most of these bacteria are commensal (ie, they coexist with the host throughout life, causing disease only under certain circumstances). For example, *Escherichia coli,* a usually benign organism commonly found in the intestines, can cause serious disease in newborns or in children with cancer. In contrast, there are certain pathogenic bacteria that almost invariably result in disease. One example is *Salmonella typhi,* which causes typhoid fever. The names of bacteria (like the names of other microbes) begin with the genus followed by the species. A genus may contain one or many species.

Bacteria are further classified according to whether they absorb a purple stain called the Gram stain (Gram positive or Gram negative), whether they prefer oxygen (aerobic or anaerobic), and whether they are round or rod shaped (coccus or bacillus). For example, *Staphylococcus epidermidis,* which colonizes the skin, is described as a Gram-positive, aerobic coccus because it absorbs the Gram stain, requires oxygen, and has a round shape. In contrast, *Bacteroides fragilis,* which is abundant in the intestines, is described as a Gram-negative, anaerobic bacillus because it does not take up the Gram stain, requires no oxygen, and is shaped like a rod.

Classifying and identifying bacteria in clinical diseases help determine the source of infection and make it possible to test the organism for susceptibility to antibiotics. Often, however, antibiotic therapy must begin before the offending microbe is identified and then must be adjusted after the organism has been cultured and tested for antibiotic susceptibility.

Mycobacteria and Spirochetes

These organisms are also at the fringe of the bacterial realm. The prototypical diseases caused by mycobacteria and spirochetes are tuberculosis and syphilis, respectively. *Mycobacterium tuberculosis* grows slowly, taking weeks to culture; *Treponema pallidum*, which causes syphilis, cannot be cultured at all. Therefore, treatment of these diseases is often based on presumptive diagnosis.

Fungi

Fungi are usually classified as yeasts (one-celled organisms) and molds (many-celled organisms with a filamentous, fuzzy appearance). Many fungi are biphasic; that is, they can assume either form, changing to fit existing conditions. Because fungi are often airborne, they frequently cause respiratory disease (see Chapter 10). One important fungus, *Candida albicans*, is not biphasic, however, but exists only as a yeast and is a frequent cause of diaper rash and thrush in infants.

Parasites

Parasites are organisms that live on or in the body, deriving sustenance from the host (see Chapter 16) . Only a few parasites are common in the United States. Among them are pinworms (*Enterobius vermicularis*) and *Giardia lamblia*, a protozoan gastrointestinal pathogen that has produced problems in day care settings. Although parasites cause relatively few problems in the United States, they pose serious and complex public health problems for other countries. Some of the most important and common diseases in the world today, including malaria and schistosomiasis, are caused by parasites.

DRUG THERAPY

In the 20th century there has been a spectacular proliferation of drugs for treating diseases. The ability to identify and routinely culture microorganisms set the stage for testing natural or synthetic compounds to combat those microorganisms. The strategy of drug therapy is nearly always the same: to interrupt a vital function of the microorganism while minimizing the effects of the drug compound on human cells. In recent years, it has been possible to perform preliminary drug testing to predict better which substances are likely to be toxic to human cells. Some therapeutic drugs are the result of systematic mass screening of compounds, and others resulted from serendipitous observations in the laboratory. An example of the latter is the story of penicillin: Accidental mold contamination of a bacterial culture killed the bacteria and led to production of the antibiotic.

The terminology of drug therapy can be confusing. The word *chemotherapy,* which most of us associate with cancer, is sometimes used to mean any kind of drug therapy. Most drug family names begin with the prefix *anti,* followed by the class of microorganisms against which the compounds act. All drugs that are used against infectious microorganisms are referred to by the generic term *antimicrobial* or, less commonly, *antiinfective* (see Table 1-1).

There is an important distinction between agents used to treat symptoms and agents used to kill germs. Management for the common cold and most viral diseases, for example, consists of treating symptoms; antihistamines may be given to relieve congestion and aspirin or acetaminophen to reduce fever. In contrast, management for strep throat and most bacterial diseases consists of eradicating the offending bacteria with antibiotics. This distinction is critical for parents and child care providers to understand because symptomatic therapy generally varies with the child's changing needs, whereas antibiotic therapy requires compliance with a specific dosage schedule.

Table 1-1 Antimicrobial Therapy for Infection

General category of infection	*General term for antimicrobial*	*Specific drug example*	*Specific infectious agent treated*	*Clinical condition*
Virus	Antiviral	Acyclovir	Herpes simplex virus	Oral or genital herpes
Bacterial	Antibiotic*	Penicillin	Group A streptococcus	Strep throat
Fungal	Antifungal	Nystatin	*Candida albicans*	Vaginal yeast infection
Parasitic	Antiparasitic†	Mebendazole	*Enterobius vermicularis*	Pinworms

*Also called antibacterial.

†Antihelmintic is a more precise term for the treatment of worms (helminths). Not all parasites are worms.

Another source of confusion for parents and child care providers is that, although many people refer to drugs by their brand names, physicians tend to use generic names (eg, penicillin) to avoid endorsing a particular brand. Awareness of this distinction can help avoid confusion in discussing drug therapy for a given illness.

Literally hundreds of different antibiotics are being used to fight bacteria, but there are relatively few medications that are active against viruses and fungi. The development of antiviral agents is hampered by the difficulty in growing and performing tests on viruses, and the drug that is most effective against serious fungal infections is often toxic to the host. The growing numbers of immunologically compromised patients who are vulnerable to certain viruses and fungi have spurred much needed development in the areas of antiviral and antifungal agents.

REFERENCES

Feigin RD, Cherry JD. *Textbook of Pediatric Infectious Disease.* 3rd ed. Philadelphia, Pa: Saunders; 1992.

Krugman S, Katz SL, Gershon AA, Wilfert CM. *Infectious Diseases of Children.* St. Louis, Mo: Mosby; 1981.

Roberts RJ. *Drug Therapy in Infants: Pharmacologic Principles and Clinical Experience.* Philadelphia, Pa: Saunders; 1984.

Stiehm ER, Fulginiti VA. *Immunologic Disorders in Infants and Children.* 3rd ed. Philadelphia, Pa: Saunders; 1989.

Chapter 2

Principles of Hygiene and Infection Control

HISTORICAL OVERVIEW

Our assumptions about how disease is caused and transmitted are different from what they were a few hundred years ago. It was once believed that disease could be caused by evil humors or bad air and that victims of plague were the objects of divine retribution. With the discovery of viruses, bacteria, and other microorganisms, however, the scientific community shifted its attention to germs and their strategies for survival. This dramatic change in focus made other insights possible. For example, it became evident that different infectious diseases had different degrees of communicability and different modes of transmission. The knowledge that malaria was carried by mosquitos and the plague by rodents and fleas made control of these devastating diseases possible for the first time in history.

The concept of contagion—the spread of disease-causing microorganisms—led to the development of antibiotics and vaccines, both of which play a critical role in controlling disease. Certain other historical developments also help control infection, although their contributions often go unappreciated. Two that are of particular relevance to the child care or school setting are the invention of the flush toilet and public sewage systems and the recognition of the importance of hand washing. Organized disposal of human waste has been attempted since ancient times, but the flush toilet provided the first reliable approach to this problem. The creation of sewage systems similarly reduced the rate of transmission of infectious diseases. Some contemporary parents look upon disposable diapers as another breakthrough in the realm of waste disposal, but the public health and environmental implications of this innovation have yet to be fully measured.

Perhaps the most important sanitary precaution is hand washing. Hand washing has been practiced in one form or another throughout history, but not until the 19th century did it become apparent that proper hand washing by medical personnel could reduce the spread of infection. Subsequent studies provided overwhelming evidence of the value of hand washing in preventing infection. The value of frequent hand washing in child care settings is almost certainly as great as it is in hospitals. In all likelihood, hand washing provides a more effective barrier to disease transmission than any of the other measures discussed in this book. Unfortunately, hand-washing practices in rest rooms, hospitals, and child care settings are far from optimal.

People practice hand washing with various degrees of thoroughness, from a ritual sprinkling of water to a 10-minute surgical scrub. To most readers, the following recommendations may be self-evident; they are not widely followed, however:

1. Rinse hands and lather with soap.
2. Wash all surfaces of hands and wrists, rubbing hands together thoroughly.
3. Rinse hands with running water.
4. Dry hands with a foot-operated air-dry machine or paper towels (communal cloth towels and, to a lesser extent, hand-operated air-dry machines may increase the risk of contamination).

Appendix B is a chart on proper hand washing, which can be reproduced for use in schools or day care centers.

HOW INFECTION IS TRANSMITTED

Despite widespread media coverage of health-related issues, misconceptions about how disease is transmitted persist. For example, many people believe they can "catch" a cold simply by leaving a window open, getting their feet wet, or experiencing a sudden change in weather. The fact is that colds are caused by microorganisms found in respiratory secretions and transmitted through the air or by direct contact. The modes of transmission for most diseases can be grouped into three general categories: respiratory (airborne), enteric (fecal–oral), and miscellaneous (direct contact, inoculation) (see Table 2-1). Isolation procedures in medical facilities are designed according to these modes of transmission. Masks are worn where respiratory transmission is possible, and gowns and gloves are used to interrupt enteric or direct-contact transmission. People with similar infectious illnesses are grouped together and apart from others, a

Table 2-1 Transmission of Human Infection

Common means of transmission	*Common examples*	*Chapter reference*
Airborne (droplet)	Viral respiratory illness, strep throat, whooping cough	Chapter 10
Enteric (fecal-oral)	Most diarrheal illnesses (salmonella, shigella, hepatitis A)	Chapter 11
Miscellaneous		
Direct contact (touch, sexual)	Herpes simplex	Chapter 14
	Impetigo	Chapter 13
Inoculation through skin (needles, transfusion, insect bites)	Hepatitis B	Chapter 11
	Some encephalitides	Chapter 9

practice known as cohorting. These general measures may be adapted for use in child care settings.

Routine Prevention of Respiratory Transmission

Everyone is at risk for acquiring most upper respiratory infections. Preventing transmission is difficult at best. Some agents that cause upper respiratory disease are airborne, and their spread may require no more than the mere presence of an infected person in the room. Fortunately, the likelihood of contagion is offset somewhat by the mild character of most childhood respiratory infections. Different respiratory infections have considerably different levels of contagion, depending in part on the size of the droplet needed to carry an infectious particle (the larger the organism, the larger the droplet). Large droplets do not stay suspended in air and therefore travel only short distances from the infected child. Two diseases that require large droplets for transmission are whooping cough and strep throat. In contrast, chickenpox and many other viral infections require only small droplets, which readily travel in air currents.

In preventing spread of respiratory illness, perhaps the factor over which educators and day care providers have the most control is containment of their own infectious secretions. Caretakers with colds should use disposable tissues and wash their hands well after blowing their noses. If possible, they should avoid contact with children who have particular difficulty with respiratory infections (eg, children with some types of congenital heart disease or with cystic fibrosis or other chronic lung conditions).

Routine Prevention of Enteric Transmission

A young child's oral habits, poor hygiene, and inability to use the toilet all contribute to the spread of enteric diseases. Enteric diseases are easier to prevent than airborne respiratory infections, however. Three preventive measures deserve special mention. First, any handling of diapers or assistance with toilets and potty chairs should be followed by hand washing (children using the potty or toilet should also wash their hands). Hand washing may be the single most effective means of interrupting enteric transmission. Second, potty chairs, if used, should be kept clean and have a removable container that can be easily sanitized. Third, diaper changes should be made in a specially designated area under specific guidelines.

The following guidelines are adapted from those prepared by the Centers for Disease Control:

- *Diapering*: Change diapers directly on paper towels, roll paper, or other disposable covering. Place this disposable covering on a surface that is:
  1. smooth, nonabsorbent, and easily cleaned (Formica® D, plastic, metal, enamel, or a diapering pad with an intact washable cover); avoid rough or porous surfaces such as tile or unsealed cement
  2. out of children's reach
  3. separate from the food preparation area
  4. within reach of a sink not used for food preparation

  Store diapers and supplies (towels, soap, bleach or disinfectant, sealable plastic bags or plastic-lined container) together in a location that is easily accessible to caretakers and out of children's reach. (Appendix C is a chart on proper diapering procedures, which can be reproduced for use in schools or day care centers.)

- *Potty Chairs*: The use of potty chairs in day care settings is discouraged. Instead, child size toilets or stepaids and modified toilet seats (which can be easily cleaned) are recommended. If these devices are not available, potty chairs which can be easily cleaned and sanitized should be used. If potty chairs are used, they should be kept in bathrooms, not in classrooms (unless in areas separated by screens or other dividers) and not in hallways where children walk. Children who are using potty chairs should not be able to reach other potty chairs, toilets, or any other surfaces likely to be covered with germs. After a child uses a potty chair:

  1. wash the child's hands
  2. empty the potty contents into the toilet

3. rinse the potty in a sink used only for this purpose, not for washing hands
4. clean and disinfect the sink
5. wash your hands

Cleaning and Disinfecting Environmental Surfaces

Disinfecting is effective only if surfaces have been thoroughly washed. Wash all surfaces with soap and water, then disinfect them with a bleach solution or a commercial disinfectant that kills bacteria, viruses, and most parasites.

To make the bleach solution, the Centers for Disease Control recommend using 1/4-cup of bleach per gallon of water. Most other authorities, however, recommend mixing 1 part bleach with 10 parts water. A spray bottle is easy to use and handy for storage. Prepare a fresh bleach solution daily. Keep this solution out of children's reach. If you are using a commercial disinfectant, consult the label or manufacturer to ascertain its effectiveness and to determine the required strength of solution.

Bathroom surfaces such as faucet handles and toilet seats should be washed and disinfected more than once a day if possible. Floors, low shelves, doorknobs, and other surfaces often touched by diapered children should be washed and disinfected weekly. Mattress covers and linen should be washed daily unless each child gets the same mattress cover every day.

Do not wash clothing that is soiled with stool. Instead, empty the stool into the toilet, being careful not to touch the toilet water with your hands. Then place the clothing in sealed plastic bags to be picked up by the child's parent or guardian at the end of the day. Always wash your hands after handling soiled clothing. Explain to parents that washing soiled clothing at the center would expose both children and staff to many disease-carrying germs.

Use only washable toys with children in diapers. Provide toys for each group so that toys are not shared among groups. Ideally, hard-surfaced toys should be washed daily, and stuffed toys should be washed weekly (more often if they are heavily soiled). Whenever possible, a toy that is mouthed by a child should be washed before other children handle it. Some establishments keep an empty container out of children's reach for storing heavily soiled toys. When time allows, these toys can be washed, disinfected, dried, and safely reused.

Keep on hand sufficient quantities of facial tissues, paper towels, and supplies for hand washing, diapering, and cleaning. Stock extra linen and mattress covers in case of accidents.

REPORTING SPECIAL INFECTIOUS DISEASE PROBLEMS

It is the responsibility of physicians, nurses, and laboratories to diagnose, treat, and report infectious diseases that are classified as reportable

Exhibit 2-1 Categories of Reportable Diseases

Report the following diseases immediately by telephone:

Botulism	Plague	Smallpox
Cholera	Poliomyelitis	Yellow fever
Diphtheria	Rabies (human)	
Measles	Rubella	

and outbreaks of any disease that may threaten public health.

Report individual cases of the following:

AIDS/HIV	Malaria	Rubeola (measles)
Amebiasis	Meningitis (specify bacterial or viral)	Salmonellosis
Anthrax	Mumps	Shigellosis
Botulism	Pertussis (whooping cough)	Smallpox
Brucellosis	Plague	Tetanus
Campylobacteriosis	Poliomyelitis	Toxic shock syndrome
Cancer	Psittacosis	Trichinosis
Cholera	Rabies	Tuberculosis
Diphtheria	Reye syndrome	Tuleremia
Encephalitis	Rheumatic fever	Typhoid fever
Hepatitis, viral (A, B, non-A–non-B, unspecified)	Rocky Mountain spotted fever	Typhus
Histoplasmosis	Rubella (congenital syndrome)	Venereal disease
Influenza	Rubella (German measles)	Gonorrhea
Legionnaires' disease		Syphilis
Leprosy		Other (specify)
Leptospirosis		Yellow fever

and any other disease that occurs in unusual numbers or circumstances or that may threaten public health (eg, epidemic diarrhea, foodborne or waterborne outbreaks, acute respiratory illness).

For schools only–Report more than 10% absence due to the following conditions (report number of cases only):

Chickenpox	Gastroenteritis	Ringworm
Conjunctivitis (pinkeye)	Impetigo	Scabies
Erythema infectiosum (fifth disease)	Influenzalike illness	Strep throat or scarlet fever
	Pediculosis (lice)	

(ie, those that have special implications for public health because of their high communicability or seriousness). Although health care personnel may have some awareness of other similar cases in the community, often educators and child care personnel are the first to find out about a communicable problem. It is therefore important that staff know which diseases have special implications for public health.

City, county, and state health departments generally provide lists of diseases that should be reported directly to them. These diseases are usually grouped in three categories (Exhibit 2-1). The first category is comprised of generally rare and extremely important diseases that should be reported immediately by telephone. A second and larger category includes common diseases that have substantial public health implications but do not require urgent reporting; the majority of reports concern diseases in this category. The third category is made up of routine infections, such as chickenpox and impetigo, for which reporting is solicited only during outbreaks. Health personnel in schools and medical offices provide important data on diseases in this category without reporting individual cases.

REFERENCES

American Academy of Pediatrics. *Report of the Committee on Infectious Diseases*. 22nd ed. Elk Grove Village, Ill: American Academy of Pediatrics; 1991.

Benenson AS. *Control of Communicable Diseases in Man*. 15th ed. Washington, DC: American Public Health Association; 1990.

Last JM, Wallace RB. *Maxcy-Rosenau-Last Public Health and Preventive Medicine*. 13th ed. Norwalk, Conn: Appleton & Lange; 1992.

Chapter 3

Immunizations

Immunization was practiced in China as early as 590 BC, when material from a smallpox pustule was instilled into the nose to prevent this disease. In 1800, the first safe vaccination against smallpox was developed in England, where it had been noted for some time that farmers who acquired cowpox were either completely protected from smallpox or had a mild, nonfatal form of the disease. Widespread vaccination programs have now eradicated smallpox throughout the world; the last case of documented smallpox occurred in October 1977. During this century, the number of available vaccines has increased dramatically, and research is constantly providing us with new or improved protection against infectious diseases.

Despite our current immunization programs, there has been a nationwide increase in vaccine-preventable diseases in recent years. Measles cases increased from an all-time low of 1,500 cases in 1983 to nearly 28,000 cases in 1990. There were 89 deaths due to measles in 1990, and 49 of these occurred in preschool-age children. The majority of deaths could have been prevented by timely immunizations. In 1990 there were also more than 1,000 cases of rubella and more than 4,000 cases of whooping cough or pertussis.

One of the reasons for this increase in vaccine-preventable diseases is the failure to immunize children at the appropriate time. Although 95% of American children are fully immunized by the time they enter kindergarten, at least 30% of all 2-year-olds in this country have not received all the currently recommended vaccines. In some inner city areas immunization rates among preschoolers are as low as 10%. There are many reasons that may contribute to our poor immunization rates, including lack of information or misconceptions about vaccines, lack of money (in 1980 it cost less than $7 to fully immunize a child at a public clinic; today, that cost has risen to more than $90), and limited access to health care in some communities.

Day care providers or directors of day care centers can work to ensure the health and safety of the children in their programs by reviewing and updating immunization records of the children regularly. If deficiencies are found, the parents of these children should be referred immediately to their child's health care provider for vaccination.

The current recommended immunization schedule for normal infants and children can be found on Table 3-1. For children with delayed immunizations, the first dose of all currently recommended age-appropriate vaccines can be administered simultaneously (eg, a 15-month-old with no previous immunizations can receive DTP/DTaP, TOPV, HbCV, HBV and MMR at the first visit; see Table 3-1 for explanations of these abbreviations). Special consideration should be given to immunization of children with human immunodeficiency virus (HIV) infection (Table 3-2).

DIPHTHERIA, TETANUS, AND PERTUSSIS

Diphtheria

Diphtheria is a severe, often life-threatening infection of the tonsils, throat, larynx, trachea, or skin caused by the bacterium *Corynebacterium diphtheriae*. The disease produces a thick, tenacious membrane that can cause suffocation if it occurs in the larynx or trachea. Certain strains of this bacterium can produce a severe inflammation of the heart muscle (myocardium). During the first quarter of this century, 200,000 cases of diphtheria occurred in this country each year, and 5% to 10% of affected individuals died. By contrast, in 1990 there were only 4 reported cases of diphtheria.

Tetanus

Tetanus (also called lockjaw), which affects approximately 60 to 90 people annually in this country, is a potentially fatal neurological disease characterized by severe, painful muscle spasms. It is caused by a toxin produced by the bacterium *Clostridium tetani* and usually results from contamination of a wound by soil, dust, or animal feces containing the bacterium. Neonatal tetanus, now rare in developed countries, results from contamination of the umbilical cord of an infant born to an unimmunized mother.

Table 3-1 Recommended Schedule for Active Immunization of Normal Infants and Children

Age	*Vaccine*
Birth	HBV*
2 months	DTP, TOPV, HbCV, HBV
4 months	DTP, TOPV, HbCV
6 months	DTP, HbCV (third HBV dose may be given at 6–18 months)
15 months	MMR, HbCV
15–18 months	DTaP, TOPV
4–6 years	DTaP, TOPV, MMR
11–12 years	MMR (unless second dose was given previously)
14–16 years	Td

HBV—hepatitus B virus vaccine
DTP—diphtheria and tetanus toxoids and pertussis vaccine
DTaP—diphtheria and tetanus toxoids and acellular pertussis vaccine
MMR—measles, mumps, and rubella vaccine
HbCV—*Hemophilus influenzae*-type b conjugate vaccine (HbCV dosing interval varies according to manufacturer; see manufacturer's insert)
TOPV—trivalent oral polio vaccine
Td—tetanus and diphtheria vaccine (reduced dose of diphtheria)

*According to option 1 (see HBV section, Table 3-4).

Pertussis

Pertussis (whooping cough), a life-threatening disease caused by the bacterium *Bordetella pertussis*, is characterized by fits of coughing that culminate in a high-pitched whoop as air is taken in (see Chapter 10). Pertussis can last for weeks or months. Before widespread use of the vaccine, 250,000 cases resulting in more than 7,000 deaths occurred annually in this country. Of these deaths, 70% occurred in children younger than 1 year. Even today, approximately 1 of every 200 infants with pertussis dies, and a significant proportion develop complications such as pneumonia, otitis media, seizures, or permanent brain damage. Today, despite an effective vaccine, pertussis continues to be a significant cause of illness and occasionally death in the United States. Between 1979 and 1988 a total of 54 deaths were directly attributable to pertussis. In 1990 there were 4,570 cases of pertussis.

In the 1970's, as a result of concern over DTP reactions, the immunization rate in Great Britain dropped from 80% to 30%. As a result, two major

Table 3-2 Recommendations for Routine Immunization of Immunocompromised Infants and Children

Vaccine	*Routine (not immuno-compromised)*	*HIV infection/ AIDS*	*Severely immuno-compromised* (not HIV related)*	*Diabetes*
DTP (DTaP/DT/dT)	+	+	+	+
TOPV	+	–	–	+
eIPV§§	use if indicated	+	+	use if indicated
MMR	+	+/consider	–	+
HbCV	+	+	+	+
Hepatitis B	+	+	+	+
Pneumococcal**	use if indicated	+	+	+
Influenzae++	use if indicated	+	+	+

§§ Enhanced-potency IPV
* Severe immunosuppression can result from congenital immunodeficiency syndromes, HIV infection, leukemia, other malignancy, treatment for malignancy, or large doses of corticosteroids
** Recommended for persons 2 years or older
++ Not recommended for infants less than 6 months of age
+ = recommended
– = contraindicated

Source: Adapted from *MMWR* (1993; 42: RR-4), April 9, 1993, Centers for Disease Control.

epidemics of pertussis occurred. Between 1977 and 1979, 102,500 cases and 36 deaths occurred in that country.

The Diphtheria, Tetanus, and Pertussis Vaccine

There are now two vaccines for diphtheria, tetanus, and pertussis. DTP is manufactured from toxins produced by the diphtheria and tetanus bacteria and from whole pertussis bacteria that have been chemically killed. This DTP vaccine has been used in the United States for more than 40 years. DTaP, a new vaccine, was licensed for use in 1991. This vaccine differs in that it contains only a portion of the pertussis organism. By including only those parts (antigens) necessary to induce immunity, many of the proteins that contributed to side effects have been eliminated from the vaccine. At this time, the DTaP vaccine has been approved for use only in children 15 months of age or older. It is anticipated that the Food and Drug Administration will approve this vaccine for use in infants as well. Because side effects to the DTaP vaccine are substantially diminished compared to those of the DTP vaccine (see Table 3-3), eventually routine vaccination of older children and adults may be possible. Those individuals

Table 3-3 Adverse Events after Pertussis Vaccine

Reaction	*Percentage of children affected*	
	DTP	*DTaP*
Redness	41	9–15
Tenderness	52	5–7
Swelling	38	5
Fever 100°–102°F	46	3–8
Fever >102°F	4	Undetermined
Crying	35	1
Irritability	34	0–22
Persistent crying	3	<1
High-pitched, unusual cry	<1	<1
Convulsions	<1	0
Collapse	<1	1

Source: Adapted with permission from Edwards KM and Karzon DT, Pertussis Vaccines, *Pediatric Clinics of North America* (1990; 37: 555), Copyright © 1990, WB Saunders.

currently are not immunized against pertussis because they usually have mild, non–life-threatening disease when they become infected and because they are more likely to experience vaccine reactions. Vaccination of this group may be important, however, because these older children and adults are frequently the source of infection in young infants, who may have severe and even fatal disease. These vaccines are injected into the thigh muscle of children 18 months of age or younger and into the arm muscle of older children.

The DTP vaccine is 70% to 90% effective in preventing pertussis after the primary immunization series. It is more than 95% effective in preventing tetanus and more than 85% effective in preventing diphtheria. The DTaP vaccine is efficacious when used as a reinforcing or booster dose (fourth and fifth doses at 15 to 18 months of age and 4 to 6 years of age) after completion of the primary series (2, 4, and 6 months of age; see Table 3-1) of DTP. The effectiveness of the DTaP vaccine in preventing pertussis and inducing immunity when given to young infants as the primary series is currently being studied.

Side Effects of the Vaccine

DTP immunization commonly causes both local and generalized reactions, including redness, swelling, and pain at the injection site, and fever, drowsiness, fretfulness, and loss of appetite. Most of these reactions can be attributed to the pertussis component of the vaccine.

Exhibit 3-1 Adverse Events after Pertussis Immunization That Usually Contraindicate Further Use of Pertussis Vaccine

Immediate, severe allergic reaction
Fever of 104.9°F (40.5°C) or greater within 48 hours
Collapse (the child becomes pale and limp) within 48 hours
Persistent, inconsolable crying for 3 hours or more or unusual, high-pitched crying within 48 hours
Convulsions within 3 days
Severe neurologic reaction (encephalopathy) within 7 days

More serious reactions can also occur. Fever of 104.9°F (40.5°C) or higher follows 1 in 330 DTP vaccinations. Seizures or episodes of collapse, in which the child becomes limp and pale, occur once in every 1,750 immunizations. Serious generalized allergic reactions or severe local reactions also occur rarely. National experts have concluded that, based on available information, vaccination with DTP has not been proven to cause permanent brain damage.

Parents and teachers should be aware that for children younger than age 7 the advantages of the DTP or DTaP vaccine far outweigh the potential risks. Routine pertussis immunization is not currently recommended for children 7 years of age and older, however, because the severity of disease caused by pertussis decreases with age and because the incidence of local or febrile reactions increases.

Children younger than 7 years who have a contraindication to pertussis immunization (see Exhibit 3-1) should receive the pediatric DT vaccine, which contains only the diphtheria and tetanus vaccine components. Because the dose given to these children would cause side effects in older children and adults, persons older than age 7 are given the Td vaccine, which contains a reduced dose of diphtheria toxoid.

A physician should be consulted before the DTP vaccine is administered to children with neurologic conditions or seizure tendencies. Current recommendations for the use of the pertussis vaccine are available from the American Academy of Pediatrics Committee on Infectious Diseases (see Appendix D).

MEASLES, MUMPS, AND RUBELLA

Measles

Measles (also known as rubeola and red or hard measles) is one of the most serious viral infections of childhood. It is characterized by a runny nose, conjunctivitis, high fever, and a rash. One in every 1,000 affected children develops inflammation of the brain (encephalitis), which can result in mental retardation, seizures, or death. Bacterial complications, such as pneumonia and otitis media, occur in 5% to 15% of infected children. In rare instances, a chronic, inevitably fatal infection of the brain (subacute sclerosing panencephalitis) develops between 4 and 14 years after measles infection.

Nationwide elimination of measles by the year 2000 is a goal set by the United States and by 32 countries in the European region of the World Health Organization. The cost of immunizing the entire world population against measles would be small compared to the cost of the disease; the success of the smallpox vaccination program proves that worldwide eradication of such diseases is possible.

Individuals born before 1956 are probably immune as a result of past measles infection. At that time, 500,000 cases of measles occurred each year. The first measles vaccine, a killed-virus vaccine, was administered in the early 1960s to approximately 800,000 people. This vaccine produced a short-lived immunity and left individuals susceptible to an atypical measles infection. When they later came into contact with the virus, they became extremely ill with high fever, headache, lethargy, unusual rash, and frequently pneumonia. This vaccine is no longer available in this country.

Soon after the killed-virus vaccine was introduced, a live-virus vaccine was made from a weakened strain of measles virus. This vaccine has been used successfully ever since. In 1983, only 1,497 cases of measles were reported in the United States. The United States has experienced a resurgence in measles cases since 1989, however, when epidemics occurred in several large urban centers. The majority of measles cases in the preschool-age group occurred in children who were vaccine eligible but had not yet received the MMR vaccine. Thus most measles cases and many deaths were potentially preventable.

In addition to preschoolers, many school-age children and young adults also developed measles during recent outbreaks. Because many of these individuals had been properly immunized, it is possible that infection occurred because of primary vaccine failure (5% of properly vaccinated children never develop protective antibody) or because of waning immunity over time. Because of these concerns a second dose of MMR is now recommended at school entry (ie, 5 years) or at entry to junior high or middle school (ie, 11 to 12 years).

Mumps

Mumps is a viral disease of childhood that commonly causes fever and headache along with swelling and tenderness of the salivary glands (particularly the parotid gland, which lies at the angle of the jaw just in front of and below the ears). More than 5,000 cases of mumps were reported in the United States in 1989.

Approximately 30% to 40% of affected individuals have no definable symptoms. Fifteen percent have a mild inflammation of the membranes covering the brain (aseptic meningitis), and 25% of postpubertal males have inflammation of the testicles. Less common complications with mumps include deafness (which may be transient or permanent), hepatitis, arthritis, and inflammation of the pancreas, breasts, thyroid, kidneys, or heart. Death from mumps is extremely rare.

Rubella

Rubella (also called German measles) is a viral disease of childhood that causes mild fever, rash, and swollen, tender lymph nodes (lymphadenopathy) behind the ears and at the back of the head and neck. Adults, particularly young women, may also have painful, swollen joints. In rare cases, encephalitis develops.

Rubella is such a mild disease in young children and adults that, were it not for its devastating effects on the fetus, vaccination programs would not be necessary. If a nonimmune woman is infected early in pregnancy, the virus can be transmitted to the fetus and cause birth defects, such as poor growth, enlarged liver and spleen, heart defects, deafness, cataracts, and mental retardation. Recent studies to determine rubella immunity indicate that 10% to 20% of young adults today are susceptible to rubella. This degree of susceptibility is similar to that seen before licensure of the rubella vaccine. Of additional concern to this large population of susceptible adults is an increase in the incidence of rubella in recent years.

In 1990, more than 1,000 cases of rubella were reported in the United States (an increase from 225 cases in 1988), and there were 10 confirmed cases of congenital rubella syndrome.

The Measles, Mumps, and Rubella Vaccine

The preferred immunization against measles, mumps, and rubella is a vaccine made from live but weakened strains of all three viruses. Optimally in the United States, children receive the first dose of the MMR vaccine at 15 months of age. If the MMR vaccine is given earlier, its effectiveness could be hampered by the immunity passed from the mother to the fetus in utero (which can last up to 12 months). Although a single injection confers lasting immunity in approximately 90% to 95% of vaccinated children, a second dose of MMR is recommended either at school entry (age 5 years) or at 11 to 12 years of age, when children enter middle school.

Side Effects of the MMR Vaccine

Rarely does the MMR vaccine cause serious reactions. Because it is a live-virus vaccine, however, it should not be given to any child with cancer, leukemia, or other disease that impairs the body's immune system. The MMR vaccine should not be given to children who are taking medication that suppresses the immune system; in these special circumstances, the vaccine can cause widespread disease. An exception to this is the child with acquired immunodeficiency syndrome (AIDS) or asymptomatic HIV infection, who should be vaccinated with MMR. These children are at risk for severe disease should they become infected with measles, and to date there have been no reports of serious reactions to the MMR vaccine in this population

Pregnant women should not receive the MMR vaccine. Vaccination of a child contact poses no risk to pregnant women or siblings with abnormal immunity, however, because the MMR vaccine viruses cannot be spread from the recipient to other persons.

Measles Vaccine

Less than 15% of vaccine recipients develop fever and rash between 5 and 12 days after immunization. The fever may exceed 103°F (39.4°C) and may persist for as long as 5 days.

Mumps Vaccine

Recipients may have fever along with swelling and tenderness of the parotid salivary gland.

Rubella Vaccine

Between 5 and 12 days after immunization, a small proportion of children will develop a rash, swelling of the glands (lymphadenopathy), and fever. Pain or swelling of the joints occurs 1 to 3 weeks after vaccination in less than 1% of young children, 1% to 3% of girls 12 years and older, and 25% to 50% of adult women. In rare cases, there may be pain, numbness, or tingling of the hands or feet.

POLIO (POLIOMYELITIS)

Polio is a viral disease that usually causes only a mild febrile illness or no symptoms at all. Infection, however, is occasionally accompanied by inflammation of the membrane covering the brain (aseptic meningitis). In 1% to 2% of cases paralytic polio develops, resulting in permanent paralysis or death. Polio vaccines, in use since 1955, have brought dramatic declines in the incidence of this potentially crippling disease. Paralytic poliomyelitis decreased from more than 18,000 cases in 1954 to fewer than 13 cases per year between 1973 and 1980. Since 1980 cases of polio in the United States either have been imported from other countries where the disease is endemic or have been associated with the administration of the live-virus oral polio vaccine.

The Trivalent Oral Polio Vaccine

The TOPV (also called the Sabin vaccine), which contains a live but weakened (attenuated) polio virus, has been used in this country since 1963. Three or four doses are required for the primary immunization series to ensure adequate protection against all three types of polio virus. The TOPV is 95% effective in producing immunity. A single booster dose before the child begins school is recommended to maintain immunity.

Along with antibodies in the blood (humoral immunity), the TOPV induces a local immune response to polio infection in the gastrointestinal tract. The live polio vaccine virus is shed in the saliva for 1 to 3 weeks and in the stools for 6 to 8 weeks after the first dose of TOPV. Virus shed in this manner can be transmitted to other children or adults who have close contact with the vaccinated child.

This is generally advantageous because these secondary contacts may thereby become immunized against polio infection. Nonimmune adults older than 18 years, however, have a slight chance (1 in every 5 to 6 million doses) of developing paralytic polio after close contact with a recently vaccinated child. There is also a small chance that the live virus can cause paralytic poliomyelitis in vaccine recipients (1 in every 8 million doses). Overall there are approximately 9 cases per year of polio vaccine–associated paralysis. Nonimmune adults may wish to be immunized with the killed polio vaccine before their children receive the TOPV. Children who receive the oral polio vaccine pose no risk to adult caretakers who have been previously immunized.

Because the TOPV is a live-virus vaccine, it can cause widespread disease in individuals who have cancer, leukemia, or other malignancy or chronic disease that weakens the body's resistance to infection. The same is true for children or adults who are taking medications that suppress the immune system (eg, steroids). These children, along with other children who have low resistance to serious infection or who live in the same household with individuals who have low resistance, should be immunized with the killed polio vaccine.

Inactivated Polio Vaccine (IPV) and Enhanced-Potency Inactivated Polio Vaccine (eIPV)

The IPV (also known as the Salk vaccine) was the first polio vaccine. It was introduced in the United States in 1955. As its name implies, this vaccine contains no live polio virus and therefore cannot cause paralytic poliomyelitis. Four separate injections of the IPV are required to produce immunity in 95% of recipients. Booster doses are recommended every 5 years for children and adolescents. No adverse side effects have been reported for the IPV.

In recent years there has been increasing interest in the development of a new killed-virus polio vaccine, one that could be given by injection during infancy and provide long-lasting immunity. There are two primary reasons for this interest. First, although the current vaccine program is largely responsible for eradicating paralytic polio in this country, there are a few vaccine recipients or contacts each year who develop paralytic poliomyelitis through contact with the live-virus vaccine. The second reason for interest in a new killed-virus vaccine is that the live-virus vaccine is not wholly effective in certain tropical countries, possibly because of inadequate immunization programs but also because of storage problems in hot tropical climates and a high incidence of gastrointestinal viral diseases, which may interfere with the body's response to the live-virus vaccine.

At this time the enhanced-potency IPV (eIPV) is licensed for use in the United States and is widely available for use in situations where a killed polio vaccine is indicated. Discussions are under way about the use of the eIPV for the first two doses of polio vaccine in the immunization schedule for normal healthy infants. This would significantly reduce the risk of vaccine-induced paralytic polio for these infants and their contacts. Potentially, the eIPV could also be combined with the DTP and other vaccines as a single injection.

TUBERCULOSIS

Tuberculosis (TB), caused by the bacterium *Mycobacterium tuberculosis,* is a disease that usually infects the lungs. In rare cases, particularly in people with AIDS or other debilitating diseases or in the very young or very old, tuberculosis may become widespread or result in meningitis.

The Bacille Calmette-Guérin Vaccine

The Bacille Calmette-Guérin (BCG) vaccine, used widely in some countries to prevent tuberculosis, is made from live, freeze-dried bacteria. It is given by injection to people considered at high risk for acquiring tuberculosis because of persistent exposure to untreated, infected individuals. This vaccine is also given to people who live in areas with high rates of tuberculosis and without health care facilities.

The BCG vaccine is not used in the United States for a number of reasons. First, there is a relatively low incidence of tuberculosis. Second, for years after vaccination, all BCG vaccine recipients have positive reactions to the Mantoux skin test for tuberculosis, making this, the most commonly used screening test, invalid. Finally, the effectiveness of the BCG vaccine has not clearly been demonstrated. In research trials conducted in the United States and elsewhere, the vaccine's effectiveness in preventing disease has ranged from 0% to 80%.

Side Effects

Between 1 and 10 of every 100 recipients of the BCG vaccine develop an ulceration at the site of the vaccination or swelling and tenderness of lymph nodes near the area. One in every million develops a bone infection (osteomyelitis). Another 1 in every million develops widespread disease or death as a result of the vaccination. Presumably some of these people have impaired immune systems.

HEMOPHILUS INFLUENZAE TYPE B

Hemophilus influenzae type b is a bacterium that causes serious, life-threatening disease in infants and children. It has been the most common cause of meningitis in children younger than 5 years and is a major cause of pneumonia, severe skin infections (cellulitis), throat infections (epiglottitis), some ear infections, joint infections (septic arthritis), and serious illness caused by bacteria in the blood stream (sepsis).

Before the availability of an effective vaccine, *H influenzae* caused 20,000 cases of severe, invasive disease in this country each year. One in every 200 children developed serious *H influenzae* disease before turning 5 years old. Each year 12,000 infections resulted in meningitis, and of these 5% to 10% caused death and up to 50% caused permanent brain damage with subsequent hearing loss, mental retardation, convulsions, or learning disabilities.

Prior to the widespread use of the vaccine, more than half of all *H influenzae* disease occurred in infants between 6 and 12 months of age; 15% occurred in children between 18 and 24 months, and 25% occurred in children 24 months or older. Certain groups of children appear to be at increased risk for *H influenzae* disease, including native Americans, children whose spleens have been damaged or removed, children with cancer or leukemia, and children in day care settings.

Hemophilus influenzae Type b Vaccine

The first vaccine against *H influenzae* type b, released in 1985, was a polysaccharide vaccine that protected children 2 years old or older but was ineffective in younger children. In 1988 an improved vaccine, the HbCV was approved for use in children at 18 months of age, and in 1990 an HbCV was licensed for use in infants beginning at 2 months of age. The vaccine is highly effective in inducing immunity (up to 100% in some studies) and has resulted in a dramatic decline in the incidence of this devastating disease. Several HbCVs are currently in use in the United States with slightly different vaccine administration schedules. All require a primary series of two to three doses with a recommendation for a booster dose at 12 to 15 months of age.

Experts recommend that all children be immunized against *H influenzae* disease beginning at their 2-month examination. Children 5 years old or younger who have not been immunized should also receive the vaccine. Physicians may recommend that certain groups of children at increased risk for *H influenzae* disease receive the vaccine beyond the age of 5 years. Children 15 months of age and older at the time of initial immunization require only one dose of the vaccine. The HbCV can be given safely at the same time as other currently recommended vaccines.

Side Effects

The HbCV is safe. It cannot cause *H influenzae* disease in recipients. Recent studies have reported side effects (redness, swelling, tenderness, and mild fever) in only 1% to 9% of vaccinated children.

HEPATITIS B

Hepatitis B virus (HBV) causes infection and inflammation of the liver. Infection may occur without symptoms or may cause jaundice, loss of appetite, nausea, malaise, arthritis, and skin rashes (see Chapter 11). HBV infection can become chronic, leading to persistent liver inflammation and damage and a lifelong risk of cirrhosis or liver cancer. Each year 250,000 to 300,000 new infections occur in the United States. Chronic infection occurs in 5% to 10% of infected adults and in a high proportion of infected neonates.

HBV can be found in semen, cervical secretions, saliva, blood, and wound exudate. Disease is transmitted sexually and in contaminated blood or blood products. It can be passed from mother to newborn at the time of birth and within families through contact of mucous membranes or abraded skin with body fluids containing infectious virus. Although HBV transmission in day care has been documented, the risk of transmission in this setting appears to be small.

Although an effective vaccine has been available for more than 10 years, the incidence of HBV infection has continued to increase. Vaccination programs have previously targeted high-risk individuals such as medical professionals, prisoners, intravenous drug abusers, and sexually active homosexual men. For approximately one third of new cases of HBV, however, no risk factor can be identified.

HBV causes more disease annually than all other vaccine-preventable diseases combined. In 1992, to reduce the incidence of disease, the Centers for Disease Control began recommending universal immunization against HBV beginning in infancy.

Hepatitis B Vaccine

The current HBV vaccine is manufactured by means of recombinant DNA technology. Unlike older vaccines, it is not produced from the serum of individuals with HBV infection. The vaccine is given in three separate doses according to one of the schedules listed in Table 3-4. The vaccine is 80% to 95% effective in preventing infection and has few adverse reactions other than soreness at the injection site.

PNEUMOCOCCAL ILLNESSES

The bacterium *Streptococcus pneumoniae* (pneumococcus) is responsible for many cases of acute otitis media. This organism is also a frequent cause of pneumonia, sinus infections, and meningitis. It is the most common cause of severe illness with bacteria in the blood stream (sepsis) in children younger than 2 years old.

Pneumococcus Vaccine

The current vaccine against pneumococcal disease is manufactured from the outer covering (capsule) of the bacteria. It is given as a single

Table 3-4 Recommended HBV Vaccination Schedules for Infants Born to Mothers Negative for HBV Surface Antigen

HBV vaccine	*Age*
Option 1	
Dose 1	Birth, before hospital discharge
Dose 2	1–2 months
Dose 3	6–18 months
Option 2	
Dose 1	1–2 months
Dose 2	4 months
Dose 3	6–18 months

HBV vaccine can be administered simultaneously with DTP, DTaP, MMR, HbCV, and TOPV. The HBV vaccine dose varies, depending on the manufacturer of the vaccine used. Please check recommendations for the vaccine used in your clinic/hospital setting.

Source: Reprinted from *MMWR* (1991; 40: RR-13), November 22, 1991, Centers for Disease Control.

injection to children older than 2 years and is not effective in younger children. Studies in children show it to be up to 37% effective in preventing pneumonia and up to 20% effective in preventing otitis media. This vaccine is currently recommended only for children in specific high-risk groups (children with sickle cell disease, nephrotic syndrome, or Hodgkin's disease or children without a functioning spleen).

Side Effects

Soreness and swelling at the site of the injection occur in one third of vaccinated children; fever greater than 99.9°F (37.8°C) occurs in 3% to 19%. Rarely is the local reaction severe or the fever greater than 102°F (38.9°C).

VACCINES AGAINST OTHER DISEASES

Meningococcus Vaccine

Vaccines against meningitis and sepsis caused by *Neisseria meningitidis* are available but not generally recommended for routine use. They are currently recommended for children with certain deficiencies of the immune system or for those traveling to foreign countries with high rates of meningococcal disease.

Influenza Vaccine

Influenza virus infections occur each year, causing anything from mild, coldlike illnesses to severe pneumonia and death. Worldwide epidemics occur periodically. The vaccine, manufactured from the killed influenza virus, can cause fever, fatigue, and muscle aches, particularly in children. Vaccination is recommended for individuals with chronic heart or lung disease, kidney disease, diabetes mellitus, sickle cell anemia, suppression of the immune system, and certain other chronic conditions. Although routine immunization of normal children is not recommended, the vaccine is safe and effective and can be given at the discretion of the physician and the parent. Influenza vaccination must be given each year because the particular strains of virus vary from year to year.

NEW VACCINES BEING DEVELOPED

Varicella (Chickenpox) Vaccine

A vaccine against varicella is being evaluated for use in normal children, and approval as a universal vaccine is expected in the future. Guidelines for use of the vaccine have not yet been completed.

Other Vaccines

Research is being conducted to develop new vaccines for cytomegalovirus infection, AIDS, rotavirus infection, Hepatitis A, and other diseases. Combination vaccines are also being developed to decrease the number of injections children receive. A vaccine that combines DTP and HbCV has already been approved for use and a Hepatitis A, B, and C combination vaccine is being studied.

REFERENCES

American Academy of Pediatrics. *Report of the Committee on Infectious Diseases*. 22nd ed. Elk Grove Village, Ill: American Academy of Pediatrics; 1991.

American Academy of Pediatrics Committee on Infectious Diseases. Acellular pertussis vaccines: recommendations for use as the fourth and fifth doses. *Am Acad Pediatr News*. 1992; 8.

Bellanti JA. Pediatric vaccinations: update 1990. *Pediatr Clin North Am*. 1990; 37:513–790.

Centers for Disease Control. Hepatitis B virus: a comprehensive strategy for eliminating transmission in the United States through universal childhood vaccination. Recommendations of the Immunization Practices Advisory Committee (ACIP). *MMWR*. 1991; 40:1–25.

Centers for Disease Control. Pertussis vaccination: acellular pertussis vaccine for reinforcing and booster use—supplementary ACIP statement. Recommendations of the Immunization Practices Advisory Committee (ACIP). *MMWR*. 1992; 41:1–10.

Centers for Disease Control. Retrospective assessment of vaccination coverage among school-aged children—selected US cities, 1991. *MMWR*. 1992; 41:103–107.

Centers for Disease Control. Rubella prevention. Recommendations of the Immunization Practices Advisory Committee (ACIP). *MMWR*. 1990; 39:1–18.

Committee on Infectious Diseases. Universal hepatitis B immunization. *Pediatrics*. 1992; 89:795–800.

Garber RM, Mortimer EA. Immunizations: beyond the basics. *Pediatr Rev*. 1992; 13:98–106.

Gindler JS, Atkinson WL, Markowitz LE, Hutchins SS. Epidemiology of measles in the United States in 1989 and 1990. *Pediatr Infect Dis J*. 1992; 11:841–846.

Sutter RW, Onorato IM, Patriarca PA. Current poliomyelitis immunization policy in the United States. *Pediatr Ann*. 1990; 19:702–706.

Chapter 4

Fever

The average body temperature is 98.6°F (37.0°C), but this can fluctuate during the day from a low of 97.0°F (36.1°C) in the morning to a high of 100.4°F (38.0°C) in the late afternoon. Body temperature that is elevated beyond this normal range is called fever. Fever is not a disease but a symptom, usually of an infectious disease.

The three areas where body temperature is commonly measured—the rectum, mouth, and armpit—give slightly different readings. Generally speaking, a fever is present if the rectal temperature is above 100.4°F (38.0°C), the oral temperature is above 100.0°F (37.8°C), or the axillary (armpit) temperature is above 99.0°F (37.2°C).

Fever is not usually dangerous or harmful unless it reaches 106°F (41.1°C) or higher, when it can have adverse effects on brain function. The body's thermostat usually keeps untreated fevers that are caused by infections below 105°F (40.6°C).

There seem to be some actual benefits of fever. A higher than normal body temperature retards the multiplication of microorganisms and inhibits their production of toxic products. Fever also enhances the body's ability to fight infection and increases the effectiveness of antibiotics.

CAUSES

The body's temperature regulator is located in a part of the brain called the hypothalamus. Fever occurs when this thermostat is set at a higher than normal value because of substances released by the body in response to infections, cancers, certain noninfectious diseases (eg, juvenile rheumatoid arthritis), certain drugs (in some individuals), and vaccines. A temporary rise in temperature can occur with exercise, environmental heat, and hot food or drink. This is not true fever, however, and the body immediately tries to lower the temperature to normal by producing perspiration, which evaporates, carrying away heat.

Contrary to popular belief, teething does not cause fever. Most fevers are due to viral illnesses, and the onset and disappearance of fever often coincide with the beginning and end of those illnesses. Most fevers that accompany viral infections range from 101° to 104°F (38.3° to 40°C) and last for 2 or 3 days. The increase in temperature does not necessarily correspond with the seriousness of the infection. Children can be perfectly comfortable and even playful with temperatures of 104°F (40°C). On the other hand, they can be quite seriously ill with an infection yet have only mildly elevated temperatures. The key to determining the seriousness of an infection is not body temperature but the way a child looks and acts.

SIGNS AND SYMPTOMS

Fevers are often accompanied by shivering or sweating. Shivering is a sign that the body is trying to elevate its temperature; sweating means that the body is trying to lower its temperature.

The common side effects of fever are generally harmless, transient, and treatable. They include mild dehydration, discomfort, a temporary disorder of mental faculties, and simple febrile seizures. A child's symptoms are more often related to the underlying illness than to the fever itself (eg, itching with a rash, cough with a respiratory infection, pain with an ear infection). Many children with mildly elevated temperatures have no other symptoms, and their illness may go unrecognized. As the temperature rises, however, the fever becomes more apparent: breathing becomes faster, the heart rate increases, and the skin appears flushed. When fever approaches 104°F (40°C), a child is likely to become listless and uncomfortable.

Febrile convulsions accompany fevers in approximately 4% of children. Uncomplicated febrile convulsions are believed to be harmless. They can occur between the ages of 6 months and 6 years, although they are most common in children between 1 and 3 years old. These convulsions usually last less than 15 minutes and are of the grand mal type. Although febrile convulsions can recur with subsequent fevers, they do not usually lead to epilepsy, and rarely do they cause brain damage. Children with recurrent febrile convulsions are sometimes given daily anticonvulsant medication until they are beyond the age of risk.

A seizure that is accompanied by fever occasionally signals meningitis and therefore requires prompt medical attention to investigate the cause and, if necessary, to initiate treatment.

TAKING THE TEMPERATURE

The main purpose of temperature taking is to determine whether a fever is present. Once this is established, it is not necessary to retake the temperature frequently unless the child feels very hot or appears to be miserable.

An electronic thermometer is recommended because it is safer, faster, and easier to use than the less expensive glass mercury thermometer. Before using the mercury (glass) type, shake it until the mercury line is below 98.6°F (37°C).

If the child is younger than 5 years, begin by taking an axillary (armpit) reading; if the temperature is above 99°F (37.2°C), take a rectal temperature.

If the child is older than 5 years, take an oral temperature.

Taking Axillary Temperatures

1. Place the tip of the thermometer in a dry armpit.
2. Close the armpit by holding the elbow against the chest for 4 minutes (or until signaled by the electronic thermometer).
3. If you are uncertain about the result, take a rectal temperature.

Taking Rectal Temperatures

1. Use a thermometer designed specifically for taking rectal temperatures.
2. Have the child lie face down on your lap.
3. Lubricate the end of the thermometer and the child's anal opening with petroleum jelly.
4. Carefully insert the thermometer about 1 inch into the rectum. Never force it.
5. Hold the child as still as possible while the thermometer is in place. Hold the thermometer between your fingers while resting the palm of the same hand cross-wise over the child's buttocks (see Figure

4-1). This both stabilizes the thermometer and allows it to move with the child, preventing sudden insertion and possible injury.

6. Leave the thermometer in the rectum for 2 minutes (or until the electronic thermometer signals).

Taking Oral Temperatures

1. Be sure the child has not recently drunk a cold or hot beverage.
2. Place the thermometer tip beside the tongue or inside the cheek.
3. Have the child hold the thermometer in place with the lips and fingers (not the teeth).
4. Have the child breathe through the nose with the mouth closed.
5. Leave the thermometer inside the mouth for 3 minutes (or until the electronic thermometer signals).
6. If the child cannot keep the mouth closed because of blocked nasal passages, take an axillary temperature.

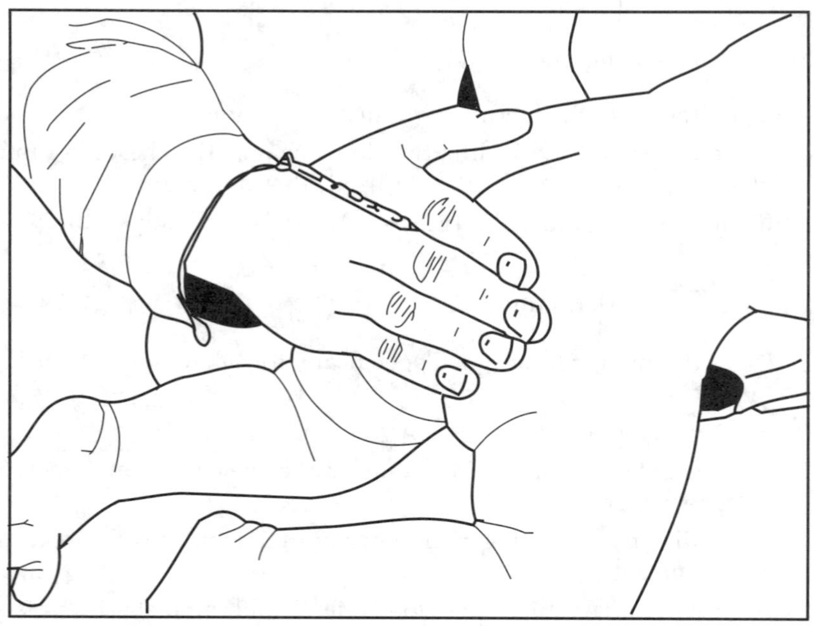

Figure 4-1 The proper technique for taking a rectal temperature

Reading the Thermometer

On a glass mercury thermometer, determine where the mercury line ends by rotating the thermometer slightly until the line appears. An electronic thermometer gives a digital reading of the temperature.

Although axillary temperatures may not be as accurate as rectal or oral temperatures, they are usually adequate for determining whether fever is present. For inexperienced persons, this technique is safer for use with young or uncooperative children than rectal temperature taking, which can result in perforations of the rectum or broken thermometers.

Forehead strips are not accurate and sometimes fail to detect fever. A hand that is accustomed to feeling children's faces is likely to detect fevers higher than 102°F, but parents, nurses, or physicians often want to know a specific temperature, which can only be obtained with a thermometer.

A new type of thermometer that reads the body's temperature from the eardrum is easy to use and seems to be quite accurate, especially in older children. A short probe is placed just inside the ear canal. The major drawback to these devices at present is their high cost.

MANAGEMENT OF FEVER

Every child with fever can be made to feel more comfortable with extra fluids, less clothing, and reduced activity. Extra fluids should be encouraged (but not forced) to help prevent dehydration. Popsicles and iced drinks are readily accepted. Because most body heat is lost through the skin, clothing should be kept to a minimum. The child should not be bundled because this can cause a rise in temperature. A light blanket can be used if the child feels cold or is shivering (has chills). Vigorous activity should be discouraged because it produces additional heat that the body must release. Quiet play, however, is appropriate.

Fever Medications

Children older than 2 months can be given one of the antifever medications listed in Table 4-1. These medications need not be given unless the fever is greater than 102°F (39°C), and even then not unless the child is uncomfortable (ie, breathing fast or feeling very hot). Most children are not uncomfortable until fever reaches 103° or 104°F (39.4° or 40°C). Although chills may cause some discomfort while the fever is rising, they often cease once the higher temperature is reached.

Table 4-1 Recommended Acetaminophen (Tylenol®, Tempra®, Panadol®, Feverall®) and Ibuprofen (Advil®, Pedia-Profen®, Medipren®, Nuprin®) Doses for Treating Fever

Child's Age	*Child's weight (pounds)*	*Drug dose*
	Acetaminophen*	
0–3 months	6-11	40 mg
4–11 months	12–17	80 mg
12–24 months	18–23	120 mg
2–3 years	24–35	160 mg
4–5 years	36–47	240 mg
6–8 years	48–59	320 mg
9–10 years	60–71	400 mg
11–12 years	72–95	480 mg
12 years and older	96 and over	325–650 mg
	Ibuprofen†	
6 months–12 years		5 mg/kg for temperature at or below 102.5°F 10 mg/kg for temperature greater than 102.5°F
12 years and older		200–400 mg

*Give every 4 to 6 hours as needed (no more than 5 doses/24 hours).
†Give every 6 to 8 hours as needed.

Acetaminophen and ibuprofen are both effective at reducing fever or pain. Aspirin, although also effective, is generally avoided in children because of the link between its use for chickenpox or influenza and Reye syndrome (see Chapter 17).

Give the correct dose for the child's age (or weight, if the child is younger than 2 years) every 4 to 6 hours, never more often than five times in 24 hours. These drugs reduce fever but usually do not bring it down to normal. Because fever fluctuates until a disease runs its course, the drug regimen often must be repeated.

Do not administer antifever drugs for more than 3 days or to infants younger than 4 months without first consulting a physician. Overdoses of these drugs are toxic. Keep them well out of children's sight and reach.

Sponging

If fever is greater than 104°F (40°C) a half hour after antifever drugs are given, sponge the child for 30 minutes in lukewarm water (sponging works much faster than immersion). Sit the child in 2 inches of water, and keep wetting the skin surface. If the fever is greater than 106°F (41.1°C), or if the child is delirious or having a seizure, sponge immediately in cool water (raise the water temperature if the child shivers). Do not expect the child's temperature to fall below 101°F (38.3°C). Do not add rubbing alcohol to the water; it can cause a coma or seizure if inhaled. Never leave a child alone in the tub; accidents can happen quickly.

Special Recommendations for Children with Febrile Seizures

If the child has a history of febrile seizures, at the onset of the fever give acetaminophen or ibuprofen at the recommended dose for 48 hours (longer if the fever persists). If the child begins to convulse, bringing the fever down as quickly as possible usually shortens the seizure. Remove clothing and apply cool washcloths to the face and neck. Sponge the rest of the body with cool water. Once the temperature drops below the seizure threshold, the seizure should stop. When the child awakens, give the appropriate dose of acetaminophen or ibuprofen.

Keep calm. The child will not be harmed by the seizure as long as breathing continues and skin color is pink (check the lips and palms in dark-skinned children). Always consult with the child's physician regarding further treatment. If the seizure lasts longer than 5 minutes or if the child is younger than 1 year or has no history of seizures, seek medical attention immediately.

When to Seek Medical Attention

Immediate medical attention is required if the child:

- is younger than 2 months
- has a temperature higher than 105°F (40.6°C)
- is difficult to awaken
- is confused or delirious
- is crying inconsolably
- is acting very sick
- is considered at high risk for a serious infection (eg, children with sickle cell disease or immune system abnormalities)
- has a seizure
- has a stiff neck
- has purple spots on the skin

- has difficulty breathing that does not improve when the nose is cleared

Less urgent but prompt medical attention is necessary if the child:

- is 2 to 4 months old
- has a temperature of 104°F (40°C), especially if the child is younger than 2 years
- has burning or pain with urination
- has ear pain
- walks with a limp (not present previously)
- complains of abdominal pain
- has fever for more than 72 hours
- has fever for more than 24 hours without obvious cause or location of infection
- has fever that ceases for more than 24 hours and then recurs

COMPLICATIONS

Fever rarely has harmful effects on the normal child. Heat stroke, however, can occur if the body is overheated and does not have a chance to dispel the heat. This can happen if a feverish child is wrapped in too much clothing, is placed near a source of heat, or is left in a car in direct sunlight without adequate ventilation. Also, excessive losses of body water due to perspiration and faster breathing can lead to dehydration (signs include strong-smelling urine and fewer wet diapers than usual). A dehydrated child is more prone to heat stroke.

REFERENCES

Fruthaler GJ. Fever in children: phobia vs facts. *Hosp Pract*. 1985; 30:49–53.

May A, Bauchner H. Fever phobia: the pediatrician's contribution. *Pediatrics*. 1992; 90:851–854.

Norris J. Taking temperatures: the changing state of the art. *Contemp Pediatr*. 1985:22–39.

Schmitt BD. Fever in childhood. *Pediatrics*. 1984; 74:929–935.

Chapter 5

Infections in Child Care Settings

Today, more than half of all mothers with children younger than 6 years are in the labor force. In 1990, 10 million children younger than 5 years were cared for by a nonparent. Of these preschool-age children, approximately 3 million were cared for by a relative or nonrelative at home, 2 million were cared for by a nonrelative in a private home, and 4 million attended organized day care centers.

The fastest growing segment of the American work force today includes the mothers of preschool-age children. This explosive growth in the employment rate of mothers with young children has brought about an unprecedented demand for child care, producing a proliferation of day care centers and family day care homes. This rapid expansion of the day care industry has outpaced our knowledge of the effects of day care on children, their families, day care personnel, and the local community (particularly with respect to the transmission of infectious diseases).

Day care regulations vary widely from state to state and, because of lack of funding, are often inadequately enforced. Many local health departments can do little more than occasionally monitor centers to ensure that minimum health and safety standards are met. Until recently there were few consistent guidelines to aid child care workers in providing safe, competent care for their young charges. In 1992, however, the American Academy of Pediatrics (AAP), in conjunction with the American Public Health Association (APHA), published *Caring for Our Children: National Health and Safety Performance Standards: Guidelines for Out-of-Home Child Care Programs*. These standards, written by experts in many fields, address issues such as environmental hygiene, personal hygiene for children and day care providers, infectious disease transmission and prevention, playground safety, and food preparation.

Day care centers present unique problems regarding hygiene and infection control. The rate of disease transmission among certain age groups has greatly exceeded that anticipated by the medical community. In fact, it was through the study of day care–related outbreaks that person-to-person transmission of certain disease-causing microorganisms (including *Hemophilus influenzae* type b, *Giardia lamblia*, and *Cryptosporidium*) was first discovered.

Although all children develop numerous respiratory and gastrointestinal (enteric) infections during the first few years of life, children in day care appear to be at significantly higher risk for certain infections, including those caused by *H influenzae* type b, cytomegalovirus (CMV), *G lamblia*, and hepatitis A virus. The day care center environment increases the likelihood that these infections, once introduced, will spread to other children, staff, or the community at large (Table 5-1).

FACTORS THAT CONTRIBUTE TO THE SPREAD OF DISEASE IN DAY CARE CENTERS

- Presence of young children in diapers
- Presence of toddlers who routinely explore their environment with their mouth and have no concept of hygiene
- Mixing of young children in diapers with other age groups
- Large group size
- High child-to-caretaker ratio
- Inadequate availability of bathroom facilities or sinks
- Staff who circulate among different age groups
- Staff who care for children as well as prepare food
- Failure of staff to observe techniques of good personal and environmental hygiene
- Lack of staff training in hygiene and infection control
- Lack of monitoring to ensure safe, healthy child care practices
- Improper disposal of tissues or soiled diapers
- Improperly designed or maintained diaper changing areas
- Use of wading pools

Diseases can be transmitted from person to person by direct contact with the infectious organism, by respiratory secretions, or by fecal–oral transmission of organisms (Table 5-2; see also chapters on specific diseases and Appendix A).

Table 5-1 Pathogens That Cause Disease among Children in Day Care Centers

	Frequency of occurrence		
Route of transmission	*Common*	*Less common to rare*	*Potential*
Respiratory	Upper respiratory pathogens (colds) Group A streptococci (pharyngitis/ tonsillitis) Varicella (chickenpox; also by direct contact) Parvovirus Influenza virus Adenovirus Respiratory syncytial virus	Meningoccous Pertussis Rubella Measles (rubeola) *Hemophilus influenzae* type b	Tuberculosis (staff to child)
Fecal–oral	Rotavirus *Giardia lamblia* Hepatitis A Enteroviruses Pinworms	*Salmonella* species *Shigella* species *Cryptosporidium* *Escherichia coli* Astrovirus Enteric adenovirus	
Direct contact	Cytomegalovirus Herpes simplex Impetigo Head lice	Epstein-Barr virus Scabies	
Blood-borne		Hepatitis B	Human immunodeficiency virus (HIV)*

*To date, no case of HIV transmission in a day care center has been documented.

Table 5-2 Communicable Diseases

Disease	*Incubation period (usual time from exposure to onset of symptoms)*	*Recommended period before reentry to school or day care (minimum exclusion period)*
Respiratory transmission		
Whooping cough (pertussis)	7–10 days	5 days after antibiotic treatment (erythromycin) is begun
Strep throat or scarlet fever	2–4 days	24 hours after antibiotic treatment is begun and fever has resolved
Mumps	12–25 days	9 days after onset of gland swelling
Measles (rubeola)	8–12 days	6 days after onset of rash
German measles (rubella)	14–21 days	7 days after onset of rash
Meningococcal meningitis	2–10 days	Until physician permits return
Hemophilus influenzae disease	Unknown, variable	Until physician permits return
Influenza	1–3 days	Until symptoms have resolved
Chickenpox or shingles (varicella zoster; spread also occurs by direct contact with rash)	7–21 days	6 days from onset of rash or until all lesions are crusted over
Tuberculosis	2–10 weeks	Until local health department determines that reentry is safe
Fecal-oral transmission		
Hepatitis A	15–50 days	7 days from beginning of symptoms or as directed by health department
Giardia lamblia infection	6–22 days	Until diarrhea is no longer present
Pinworms	3–6 weeks	After treatment
Enteroviruses	1–3 days	Until diarrhea is no longer present
Rotavirus	1–3 days	Until diarrhea is no longer present

Table 5-2 continued

Disease	*Incubation period (usual time from exposure to onset of symptoms)*	*Recommended period before reentry to school or day care (minimum exclusion period)*
Salmonella infection	6–72 hours	Until local health department determines that reentry is safe (usually until acute illness has resolved and diarrhea is no longer present)
Shigella infection	1–7 days	Until local health department determines that reentry is safe (usually after antibiotic course is completed and/or stool cultures are negative)
Transmission by direct contact		
Impetigo	7–10 days	24 hours after antibiotics are begun
Scabies	4–6 weeks in people who have not been infected previously; 1–4 days in people who have been infected	Day after treatment is completed
Lice	Eggs hatch in 1 week	Day after treatment is completed
Cytomegalovirus	Unknown	Exclusion is not recommended even though virus can be spread as long as CMV is present in urine or saliva
Herpes simplex gingivostomatitis	3–5 days	Children who do not have control of oral secretions should be excluded until mouth sores have cleared; children with mild illness who are in control of oral secretions may not require exclusion
Infectious mononucleosis	10–50 days	Until symptoms have resolved and child can participate in center activities
Purulent conjunctivitis	1–3 days	24 hours after antibiotic treatment is begun

DISEASES SPREAD BY RESPIRATORY SECRETIONS

Viral Upper Respiratory Infections (Colds)

Upper respiratory infections (see Chapter 10) are the most common cause of illness in children, representing 60% to 75% of all acute illnesses. Normal children may experience between 6 and 10 respiratory illnesses in a single year; the highest incidence is among children between 6 months and 1 year of age. Children in day care have half again as many respiratory infections during the first year of life as children who are cared for at home. These infants also have up to three times as many acute illnesses with fever. Although children who enter day care in infancy have a higher rate of illness during the first year of life, in subsequent years they appear to have a lower rate of respiratory illness than their peers who are cared for at home. Presumably this decreased rate of illness is due to a gradually acquired immunity to many respiratory diseases.

Viral upper respiratory infections do not respond to antibiotic therapy. Therefore, management consists primarily of treating those symptoms that are particularly bothersome to the child (such as nasal congestion, which makes breathing difficult; cough, which interferes with sleep; or fever, which causes discomfort and irritability). Because all medications may have side effects, caretakers and parents should be careful not to overmedicate children who have colds.

Children with uncomplicated respiratory illnesses (and possibly mild febrile illnesses as well) need not be excluded from day care if they appear to feel well, behave normally, and are able to participate in usual daily activities. The child with fever who appears to be uncomfortable, is less active than usual, has a poor appetite, or is fussy or irritable, however, should be excluded from day care until these symptoms resolve. A child who has these symptoms but no fever may also require exclusion, depending upon the severity of the symptoms and the ability of the center to provide the kind of care the child requires.

Otitis Media

Otitis media (see Chapter 8), the most frequent complication of upper respiratory infections, accounts for more visits to physicians' offices than almost any other disease. Children in day care have from two to four times as many episodes of otitis media as children who are cared for at home.

Acute otitis media usually requires treatment with antibiotics. Affected children may experience significant pain requiring antipain medication, such as acetaminophen, for several days. Research has indicated that decongestants and antihistamines are ineffective in preventing otitis media or hastening the resolution of the illness.

Otitis media is not contagious. Children with otitis media do not require exclusion from day care if they are able to participate normally in daily activities or if the day care center has the staff and facilities to care for a sick child.

Hemophilus influenzae Type b

Despite its name, *Hemophilus influenzae* is a bacterium and is not related to the viruses that cause the yearly winter outbreaks of influenza. It causes disease almost exclusively in children younger than 5 years and was a common cause of meningitis in children. It also causes pneumonia and severe infections of the skin (cellulitis), throat (epiglottitis), joints (septic arthritis), and blood stream (bacteremia). Before widespread use of the vaccine, 20,000 cases of serious *H influenzae* disease (including 12,000 cases of meningitis) occurred in this country each year. Sixty percent of *H influenzae* disease occurred in children younger than 18 months, with the highest incidence among children between 6 and 12 months old. Since universal immunization of all infants was initiated in 1990, *H influenzae* has decome a relatively uncommon disease.

Certain groups of children appear to be at increased risk for acquiring *H influenzae* disease. These include native Americans, African-Americans, children with sickle cell disease and those without spleens, children with certain malignancies or immune deficiency syndromes, and unimmunized children attending day care.

Signs and Symptoms of H influenzae *Disease*

- Meningitis: fever, headache, irritability, lethargy, poor feeding, and stiff neck (suspected meningitis requires immediate medical attention!)
- Cellulitis: fever and irritability; skin that is reddish or purple, swollen, tender, and warm, usually on the cheek or around the eye
- Septic arthritis: fever, refusal to walk or to use a joint that may be extremely tender, swollen, red, and warm
- Epiglottitis: fever; rapid onset of severe sore throat; refusal to eat or drink; drooling; ill, anxious appearance; high-pitched, crowing noises as swelling obstructs the airway; sitting or leaning forward to breathe more easily (epiglottitis requires emergency medical treatment!)
- Pneumonia: fever, cough, and increased rate of breathing
- Bacteremia: fever, irritability, and fatigue

Management and Prevention

If a case of *H influenzae* disease is diagnosed in a day care center, all parents should be notified of the exposure, informed of the risk of spread, and advised regarding signs and symptoms of illness to look for in their own children. The local health department should be consulted for assistance and recommendations regarding management.

In a group day care setting, there is a risk of subsequent (secondary) cases of *H influenzae* disease among classmates of the infected child. To prevent the spread of disease, the antibiotic rifampin is often recommended for household and day care contacts. Rifampin appears to decrease the spread of *H influenzae* disease and is relatively safe, causing few adverse effects. Some authorities, including the US Public Health Service Advisory Committee on Immunization Practices, recommend that rifampin prophylaxis be used whenever a case of serious *H influenzae* disease (meningitis, bacteremia, etc) occurs in a day care facility where children younger than 2 years have been exposed. This recommendation is somewhat controversial. The AAP has published guidelines that suggest rifampin prophylaxis of day care contacts only if there are children present who are younger than 2 years with contact of 25 hours per week or more. The AAP does not recommend rifampin in facilities where all contacts are older than 2 years unless more than one case of *H influenzae* disease has occurred. Authorities agree that, when two or more cases of *H influenzae* disease occur within a 60-day period, rifampin should be administered to all children and day care personnel in the classroom attended by the infected child.

For rifampin to be effective in preventing the spread of disease, all children and staff in the classroom must receive the antibiotic promptly. It is important that caretakers as well as children receive rifampin because adults can carry the bacteria in their nasopharynx and transmit it to susceptible children.

Children who have been exposed to *H influenzae* should be observed for signs and symptoms of illness. The period of observation should extend for at least 60 days from the last exposure. Signs of illness or fever should be reported immediately to the parents with the recommendation that the child be evaluated by a physician.

The H influenzae *Vaccine*

Hemophilus influenzae conjugate vaccines have been approved for use in infants beginning at 2 months of age since October 1990 (see Chapter 3). These vaccines are safe, have few side effects, and effectively prevent *H influenzae* infection in infants completing the multidose schedule. Since routine immunization of infants was initiated, the incidence of invasive *H influenzae* disease in children younger than 2 years has decreased by more than 90% in some areas of the United States. Because children in day care are at increased risk of exposure to *H influenzae*, it is imperative that day care personnel ensure that all children attending the facility are appropriately immunized.

DISEASES SPREAD BY DIRECT CONTACT

Cytomegalovirus

Cytomegalovirus (CMV), a member of the herpesvirus family, is transmitted through close personal contact with body fluids of infected individuals (urine, saliva, semen, mucus from the uterine cervix, and breast milk). After infection, the virus may be excreted for a period of weeks to months. Some congenitally infected children (infected before birth) excrete the virus for years (see Chapter 14).

CMV infection is common among young children who are cared for in groups. Overall, 20% to 60% of children in any given day care center can be expected to have CMV in their urine or saliva. In fact, among toddlers in day care centers, the incidence of CMV excretion is often greater than 50% and may be more than 90%. Our own experience has confirmed that CMV infection occurs frequently even in day care centers with good hygienic practices. Transmission is particularly common as young children become more mobile, curious, and sociable and as they begin to explore the world by putting everything into their mouths. On average, children who become infected with CMV in day care excrete the virus for more than 7 months in saliva and for more than 1 year in urine. These children can, therefore, be a source of infection for prolonged periods of time. The virus can also persist in saliva on an environmental surface for up to 2 hours and thus could be transmitted by shared mouthing toys, eating utensils, or drinking glasses. CMV can also survive for many hours in a urine-soaked disposable diaper, making this a possible source of transmission in the day care center.

Sooner or later, nearly everyone is infected with CMV. Infection usually occurs without symptoms and is rarely of consequence for the infected child or adult. Occasionally, CMV infection can cause symptoms resembling those of infectious mononucleosis with fever; swollen, tender lymph nodes; and malaise. The groups at risk for severe disease or serious complications after CMV infection are individuals whose immune systems are impaired [such as those with acquired immunodeficiency syndrome

(AIDS)] and pregnant women who are not already immune to CMV. If CMV infection occurs in a nonimmune pregnant woman, there is a small chance that the developing fetus will be severely damaged by the virus (see Chapters 14 and 17).

The prevention of all CMV transmission among children in day care is not practical and may not be desirable. Early infection induces immunity and, in girls, eliminates the risk of acquiring the virus for the first time during pregnancy. As with all communicable diseases, however, good hygiene may reduce the risk of transmitting CMV infection. Environmental surfaces such as table tops and toys mouthed by young children can be disinfected with a solution of 1 part chlorine bleach to 10 parts water. Nonimmersible items can be air dried for several hours before being reused. Child care providers should wash their hands with warm, soapy water after intimate contact with infants or young children, particularly after diaper changes or contact with saliva or nasal secretions. The use of disposable gloves for diapering is not required but has been recommended by some experts. Diapers should be disposed of in suitable containers.

Because CMV infection is common among children in group care settings, it is neither necessary nor practical to exclude from day care a child who is excreting CMV. Congenitally infected, handicapped infants should not be excluded from center-based programs and should continue to receive the educational and therapeutic services they require. Although congenitally infected children may excrete CMV in their urine and saliva for years after birth, isolation of these children is not warranted. The issue of prevention of CMV transmission to adult caretakers or parents is complicated and is addressed more fully in Chapter 6.

Herpes Simplex

Herpes simplex virus, transmitted by direct contact with an infected individual, produces a wide spectrum of disease (see Chapters 6 and 14). The incubation period is usually from 2 to 5 days. Affected individuals are considered contagious while active, blisterlike (vesicular), or ulcerated skin lesions are present in the mouth, on the skin, or on the genitals. Recurrent herpes infections, such as the cold sore, are common. Affected individuals are able to transmit the herpes simplex virus to others during these recurrences.

Although primary (first) infection with this virus commonly occurs without symptoms, some children develop a gingivostomatitis, which usually occurs during infancy and is characterized by fever, irritability, and an ulcerated, blisterlike rash on the inside of the mouth and throat. The gums become red and swollen and may bleed easily. The lymph nodes in the neck become swollen and tender. Although symptoms can be severe, more often they are so mild that the infection is never brought to the attention of a physician and therefore never diagnosed.

Herpes simplex infections may involve the eye (causing severe conjunctivitis) or any skin surface. Children with eczema are at risk for developing herpes infection of eczematous skin surfaces that are exposed to the virus.

The only children at risk for severe herpes infections are infants younger than 1 month, children with lowered resistance to infection (immunodeficiency), and children with extensive skin disease such as eczema (atopic dermatitis).

Children with primary or recurrent herpes infection of the mouth or lips who do not have control of their oral secretions (drooling, spitting, or frequent hand- or object-to-mouth behavior) should be excluded from day care until their symptoms resolve and the vesicles have crusted (usually 4 to 5 days after they appear). Children with recurrent herpes infection of the skin should be excluded (until the lesions have crusted) only if the vesicles involve an area of the body that cannot be adequately covered by clothing, a bandage, or other appropriate dressing. When the vesicles are crusted over or are not present, there is no risk of infection for caretakers or other children who have close physical contact with the affected child.

Older children or adult caretakers with recurrent oral herpes may attend school or day care if they practice good hygiene (eg, performing proper hand washing, not touching their sores, and not kissing or engaging in similar close contact with others). Day care workers with active herpes lesions of the mouth or skin should avoid contact with infants younger than 1 month. Adults with recurrent genital herpes presumably do not pose a risk for the children under their care. Genital herpes is a sexually transmitted disease that is unlikely to be acquired or transmitted in a child care environment. If herpes infection recurs on the body, arms, or legs, clothing that covers these areas will decrease the risk of transmission.

There are times when it is desirable for a child with active, recurrent herpes lesions to continue to receive center-based care. For example, children receiving intensive therapy for hearing, visual, or physical deficits should attend sessions provided that they are isolated from other young children, that the sores are covered with clothing or a bandage, and that caretakers use gloves or gowns if direct contact with the sores is unavoidable.

DISEASES SPREAD BY FECAL-ORAL TRANSMISSION

Many diseases can be spread among groups of children through contact with feces from an infected individual. These diseases pose a particular problem in day care centers that accept infants and young children in diapers. The opportunity for transmission of disease is great among toddlers, who have poor hygiene but excellent mobility. Careful hand washing is important for both children and staff. Also, care must be taken to disinfect changing tables and to dispose of soiled diapers properly.

One type of illness spread by the fecal-oral route is infectious diarrhea (see Chapter 11). This disorder is particularly prevalent in large day care centers and in centers that accept young infants and toddlers in diapers. Infection spreads rapidly when loose or liquid stools run down a child's legs or soak through clothing and contaminate caretakers' hands or environmental surfaces (floors, cribs, toys, clothing, doorknobs, etc). Good hygiene is essential in preventing transmission of diarrheal disease to other children. In fact, frequent, thorough hand washing alone can reduce the incidence of diarrhea in day care centers by as much as 50%.

Giardia lamblia

Giardia lamblia (see Chapter 16) is a parasite that can cause diarrhea, abdominal bloating, gas, poor appetite, weight loss, and vomiting. Infection can also occur without symptoms. It is now recognized as a leading cause of diarrheal illness in child care environments. Person-to-person transmission of *G lamblia* was first recognized during outbreaks of diarrhea among children in day care centers. Studies have found that, even in centers without an increased incidence of diarrhea, as many as 26% of children are asymptomatic carriers of *G lamblia*. The infection frequently spreads (usually by the contaminated hands of children or care providers) to family members and the community at large.

When a case of *G lamblia* is identified in the day care center, the local health department should be notified. Parents of other children in the center should also be notified of the exposure. All symptomatic children, day care providers, and family members (ie, those with diarrhea) should be evaluated to determine whether *G lamblia* cysts are present in stool, and those infected with the organism should be treated. Infected individuals with diarrhea should be excluded from day care until the diarrhea resolves. Infected but asymptomatic individuals can also spread the disease to others. Treatment or exclusion of these children has not been shown to be effective in stopping the spread of disease, however. Therefore, only individuals with symptoms of infection need to be screened for the organism and treated if positive. Those found to be infected should be treated with an antiparasitic drug (furazolidone, metronidazole, or quinacrine). After the diarrhea has resolved, the child may return to day care.

Salmonella

Salmonella species are bacteria that rarely cause outbreaks of diarrhea among children in day care centers. Salmonella infection can occur without symptoms or with high fever, severe cramping, and loose stools that contain blood and mucus. Young infants, children with sickle cell disease, and other children with lowered resistance to infection can develop severe disease involving the blood stream (bacteremia), bones (osteomyelitis), or the coverings around the brain (meningitis).

Salmonella organisms can be spread from person to person (infected children and adults can excrete the organism in their stools for weeks or months). Transmission can also occur through contaminated poultry and other livestock, raw milk, and pet turtles.

Antibiotic treatment is usually reserved for children who are at risk for severe, overwhelming disease. When antibiotics are used for uncomplicated salmonella diarrhea, the bacteria may be shed in the stools for a longer than usual period of time.

If salmonella infection is identified in a day care center, it should be reported to the local health authorities, who will assist in managing the outbreak. Parents of other children attending the center should also be notified of the exposure. Infected children with diarrhea should be excluded from the day care center until the diarrhea ceases. Asymptomatic contacts need not have stools cultured.

Shigella

Shigella species are also bacteria that can cause outbreaks of diarrhea in day care centers. Infection can occur without symptoms or with only loose, watery diarrhea. Shigella infection can also cause severe illness with high fever, abdominal cramping, headache, watery stools containing blood and mucus, and occasionally convulsions or significant body water loss (dehydration). Girls with shigella infections may also develop vaginitis (see Chapter 12).

Infection with shigella organisms is more common among children who wear diapers, but the bacteria can spread to adult day care center staff, household members, and the community at large.

If shigella infection occurs in the day care center, the local health department should be consulted for recommendations and assistance in preventing or managing an outbreak. Parents of other children in the day care center should be notified of the exposure.

Stool cultures for the shigella organism should be performed for all symptomatic children, staff in the classroom, and members of the infected child's household. All individuals with confirmed shigella infection should receive antibiotic treatment and be excluded from day care until the diarrhea has resolved.

Rotavirus

Rotavirus, a common infection in young children attending day care, typically causes diarrhea, vomiting, and low-grade fever and occasionally respiratory symptoms such as cough and runny nose. Transmission occurs through contact with feces and possibly respiratory secretions. This virus can cause particularly severe disease in children younger than 2 years and can lead to dehydration requiring medical care.

Usual procedures to interrupt transmission of enteric infections should be implemented, including careful, monitored hand washing and exclusion of children with diarrhea until the diarrhea ceases. Vaccines against rotavirus are currently being tested.

Other Causes of Diarrhea in Day Care Centers

Several other bacterial and parasitic organisms can cause isolated cases or outbreaks of diarrhea in day care centers. Outbreaks of diarrheal disease due to cryptosporidium parasites have occurred in several day care centers across the country. In 1993, the city of Milwaukee experienced one of the largest water-borne disease outbreaks in history, proven to be cryptosporidiosis. Infection with this organism was once believed to occur only in immunosuppressed individuals. Children with cryptosporidiosis usually have mild, self-limited diarrheal disease without fever. No satisfactory treatment is available. Other causes of diarrhea include infection with astrovirus, calicivirus and certain strains of *Escherichia coli*.

Careful personal and environmental hygiene will result in less diarrheal disease in day care facilities. To interrupt transmission of organisms that cause diarrhea, staff should receive specific training in disease transmission and hygienic techniques for themselves, the children, and the environment. Frequent hand washing at appropriate times for staff and children (see below, Guidelines for Preventing Disease Spread in Day Care

Centers) should be enforced and monitored at least weekly. The center should exclude ill children until the diarrhea has resolved and the stools can be adequately contained within the diaper. Usually, asymptomatic children (those without diarrhea or signs of illness) who shed diarrhea-causing organisms in the stool do not need to be excluded or receive treatment unless specifically directed by the health department.

Hepatitis A

Hepatitis A (infectious hepatitis), a viral infection that can damage the liver, poses a major potential health risk in day care centers. The chances of hepatitis A being introduced into a day care center depend upon the incidence of the disease in the community and the number of children enrolled in the center. Once the disease is introduced, the likelihood of spread depends primarily on whether children in diapers are present.

Several communitywide epidemics have been linked to outbreaks in day care centers. Therefore, control of disease within these centers may help limit the spread of hepatitis A into the community. In Phoenix, Arizona, aggressive management programs during day care outbreaks have resulted in a 75% decrease in community disease as well as a substantial reduction in the extent of hepatitis outbreaks in day care centers.

Young children with hepatitis A infections often have no symptoms or only mild, nonspecific symptoms such as fever, vomiting, diarrhea, loss of appetite, and fatigue. Only 5% to 10% of toddlers or preschoolers have dark, tea-colored urine and jaundice (a yellow color to the skin and eyes), indicating liver damage. In contrast, 75% of affected adults are visibly jaundiced. The disease often goes unrecognized in day care centers until staff or family members become ill and have noticeable jaundice. By the time an outbreak is recognized, the disease is often already widespread.

There is no effective treatment for hepatitis A. Most affected children and adults have only mild disease and recover without consequences, however. Management is aimed primarily at preventing disease (through good hygiene) and controlling outbreaks. Immune globulin (Ig, a blood product that contains antibodies) is used in certain situations to prevent the spread of infection. The local health department should be notified any time a case of hepatitis A occurs in day care children, staff, or household members. Parents should also be notified of the exposure and of signs and symptoms to observe for in their child or other family members.

If hepatitis A develops in an employee or child in a center with only children older than 2 years of age or only those who are toilet trained, all staff members who have contact with the infected child and all children in the same classroom as the infected child should receive Ig. In centers with children younger than 2 years or children in diapers, the following recommendations apply:

- If hepatitis A develops in a single child or employee of the center or in household contacts of center children from two different families, all children and employees at the center should receive Ig.
- All children or employees who join the center during the 6 weeks after the last case should also receive Ig.

If more than 3 weeks have passed before a hepatitis A outbreak is recognized, or if three or more families of center children have reported a case of hepatitis A, the disease is probably already widespread. In this case, Ig prophylaxis should be considered for all center children and employees and all household contacts of center children in diapers.

These recommendations may change periodically, so that providers should consult with local health authorities for the most current information. Children or staff who are ill with hepatitis A should be excluded from day care until 1 week after the onset of symptoms and until jaundice has resolved.

DISEASES SPREAD BY BLOOD OR BLOOD-CONTAINING BODY FLUID

Hepatitis B

Hepatitis B virus (HBV) infection causes inflammation of the liver (see Chapters 3 and 11). Infection may occur without symptoms or may cause serious illness with jaundice, pale stools, dark urine, loss of appetite, and occasionally death. Although most infected adults become noticeably jaundiced, this is rare in young children. In some cases infection may become chronic. Individuals with chronic HBV infection are at risk of developing cirrhosis or liver cancer in later life.

HBV is transmitted sexually or by blood or blood-containing body fluids. The virus can be found in blood, semen, cervical secretions, saliva, and wound discharge. Although there have been rare reports of HBV transmission in day care settings, this appears to be uncommon.

Current recommendations for the universal vaccination of all children will substantially diminish the risk of HBV transmission. Children with chronic HBV infection can attend day care unless they have behavioral (unusually aggressive behavior such as biting and scratching) or medical (bleeding problems or generalized dermatitis) risk factors. Admission should be assessed on an individual, case-by-case basis by the child's physician, the center director, and public health authorities. The center director and primary caregiver should be informed about the HBV status of any HBV carrier attending the center. Regular reassessments of the child's medical condition and behavior should be performed.

Because children with undiagnosed or unreported chronic HBV infection undoubtedly attend day care, universal precautions should be used whenever contact with blood or body fluids is anticipated (see below, Guidelines for Preventing Disease Spread in Day Care Centers). HBV can potentially be transmitted by saliva, although infectivity by this route is low. The virus can also exist on environmental surfaces for extended periods of time. Therefore, hygienic measures should be employed to limit environmental contamination with saliva.

Although bites are an uncommon means of HBV transmission, the potential for spread by this route exists. If a known chronic HBV carrier bites another child, hepatitis B immune globulin (HBIG) prophylaxis is recommended for the victim. If a known chronic HBV carrier is bitten by another child, HBIG is recommended for the biter if the biter has an open sore or cut on the lips or mouth or if there is more than a small amount of bleeding from the bite. In either event, the parents of the biter and the victim should be notified and the health department representative and/or physician consultant contacted for recommendations.

Human Immunodeficiency Virus

Infection with HIV can result in a spectrum of illnesses ranging from asymptomatic infection to overwhelming disease involving many body organs and ultimately resulting in death. AIDS, the most commonly recognized disease state produced by this virus, results from the failure of the body's immune system to protect against disease. Individuals with AIDS may have severe or unusual infections; certain cancers; enlargement of lymph nodes, liver, and spleen, poor growth; chronic diarrhea; kidney or eye disease; and progressive disease and deterioration of the nervous system.

HIV is transmitted sexually, by blood or blood products, or through contact with blood-containing body fluids. The virus can be found in semen, cervical secretions, blood, wound discharge, breast milk, and several other body fluids. High-risk groups include homosexual or bisexual men and their sexual partners, intravenous drug abusers, recipients of blood or blood products (eg, hemophiliacs) before widespread testing of the blood supply for HIV, and children born to women with one or more of these risk factors. Transmission by casual contact within the family (even with sharing of food, utensils, and toothbrushes) has not been demonstrated.

To date, there has been no documented case of HIV transmission in a day care setting. Large studies to address specifically the issue of risk of transmission in out-of-home day care have not been performed, however.

Children with HIV infection can be safely admitted to day care provided that their health, neurologic development, behavior, and immune status are appropriate. The decision regarding admission of an HIV-infected child to a particular day care situation should be made on a case-by-case basis by qualified individuals, including the child's physician, the day care center director, and the child's family. Children who exhibit particularly aggressive behavior (such as biting or scratching) or who have open skin lesions should not be admitted to day care. Children with severely compromised immune systems may be at great risk from diseases acquired in a day care setting.

The day care center director and primary day care provider should be notified of any child in their care with HIV or any disease or disorder that impairs the immune system and makes the child more susceptible to infection. The provider will need to notify the parents of an immunodeficient child immediately should exposure to certain diseases (such as chickenpox or measles) occur. The child should be reassessed periodically to determine whether day care placement continues to be appropriate.

Undiagnosed or unreported HIV-infected children are currently attending out-of-home day care. Staff should use universal precautions (see below, Guidelines for Preventing Disease Spread in Day Care Centers). Environmental hygiene should minimize contamination of environmental surfaces with body fluids.

GUIDELINES FOR PREVENTING DISEASE SPREAD IN DAY CARE CENTERS

- Hand washing is the most important means of controlling infection. Staff and children should wash their hands upon arrival at the center, after using the toilet or changing diapers or soiled pants, after assisting with toilet use, after wiping a child's or their own runny nose, after handling animals, before serving or eating food, and any time hands may be contaminated with a body fluid.
- Staff shall adopt universal precautions to protect themselves and others from potential exposure to blood, blood-containing body fluids, or discharge from an injury or sore. Hand washing after exposure to

these fluids should be enforced. Avoid contact with these fluids by wearing gloves. Either single-use disposable gloves or heavy, reusable utility gloves are acceptable. Gloves designated for single use should be discarded after use and not washed and reused. Heavy, reusable gloves should be washed (while worn) with soap and water and then disinfected in a bleach–water solution and hung to dry. Spills of blood or blood-containing body fluids should be cleaned up and surfaces then disinfected with a bleach–water solution (1/4 cup of bleach to 1 gallon of water or 1 part bleach to 10 parts water). Gloves should be worn during clean-up. To ensure compliance with these recommendations, gloves should be available in an easily accessible area for staff. Personnel supervising children on a playground should carry disposable gloves (and gauze pads in a plastic bag) so that they are prepared to handle any traumatic injuries with bleeding that may occur.

- The diaper changing table should be cleaned and disinfected after each use. Mouthed toys should also be disinfected after each use. Toys that are frequently handled by infants and toddlers should be cleaned and disinfected daily. Stuffed animals intended for communal use are discouraged.
- Different age groups should be kept separate, even on the playground or during the early morning or late afternoon hours, when there are fewer children present. This is particularly important if there are young children in diapers.
- Food preparation centers should be located well away from child care areas. Where circumstances permit, the person who prepares the food should not also be a care provider.
- An area should be set aside for segregating sick children until their parents can pick them up.
- Play areas should be cleaned frequently, floors should be vacuumed or swept and mopped daily with a sanitizing solution, and bathrooms should be disinfected more than once a day. Food and litter should be removed as they accumulate.
- Soiled clothing should be returned to parents daily in a plastic bag for laundering (at home, not at the center).
- Diapers and waste materials (bandages, tissues, etc) contaminated with blood or other body fluid should be disposed of in a plastic bag that is securely closed.

- Each child should have a separate cot or mat for naps; bed linens should be changed at least weekly (daily for infants). Crib mattresses and furniture should be cleaned and disinfected weekly.
- Exclusion policies should be communicated to parents when the child is enrolled (see Exhibit 5-1).
- Parent information handouts (see Appendix A) should be distributed as the need arises to inform parents of actual or potential disease outbreaks, symptoms to look for in their children, and instructions about what action to take if symptoms develop.
- The day care center should establish a health professional liaison in the community to provide information, answer questions, and assist with disease management.
- Day care staff should be familiar with state regulations regarding illness in day care, reportable diseases, and individuals or groups who can provide assistance with management and prevention of disease outbreaks.
- Care providers should be instructed in the routes of disease transmission, personal and environmental hygiene, and the use of universal precautions.

EXCLUDING SICK CHILDREN FROM DAY CARE

Sick children may be excluded, isolated, or cohorted (grouped, see Chapter 2). The appropriate alternative depends on the nature of the disease and on available staff and facilities. During certain outbreaks, it may be feasible to cohort all ill children apart from the well children. If only one or two children are ill, however, the cost of isolating them with a staff member is prohibitive. For this reason, most day care centers must have exclusion policies to prevent the spread of disease.

Sick child exclusion guidelines that are too stringent can be an enormous burden for working parents, who may lose pay (or even their jobs) if too many work days are spent at home caring for sick children. This, of course, can place a strain on the relationship between day care personnel and parents. The phone call that informs parents that they must leave work to pick up a sick child is often as difficult for the day care provider to make as it is for the parent to receive. On the other hand, lax standards can cause increased illness among staff, children, their families, and the community. Day care personnel must remember that caring for a sick child is ultimately the parents' responsibility.

Exhibit 5-1 Exclusion Guidelines for Day Care Centers

Mildly ill children who can participate normally in the activities of the center need not routinely be excluded.

Determine the following:

1. Can the child participate normally in the usual activities of the center?
2. Does the child require more intense care and attention than the staff can reasonably provide?
3. Does the child have a condition or disease that poses a potential risk to either the child or others?

Children with the conditions listed below should be excluded until the symptom/condition has resolved or until evaluation by a medical professional determines that the child can return to the center:

1. Fever (oral, 101°F or greater; rectal, 102°F or greater; axillary, 100°F or greater) plus:
   - behavior change (irritable, cranky, restless, listless) and/or
   - symptoms of illness
2. Evidence of severe illness: lethargy; unusual sleepiness; irritability; prolonged crying; inconsolability; obvious discomfort; labored, difficult or rapid breathing; extreme or uncontrollable coughing; wheezing; poor appetite
3. Rash associated with other signs of illness, fever, or change in behavior
4. Purulent conjunctivitis (pink eye) with pus accumulation
5. Diarrhea; increased number and water content of stools that cannot be contained within the diaper
6. Vomiting; more than twice in a 24-hour period
7. Herpes gingivostomatitis; mouth sores or ulcers if the child cannot control his or her saliva
8. Children with certain specific infections: pertussis or whooping cough, strep throat, head lice or scabies, chickenpox, tuberculosis, impetigo, mumps, measles, rubella, hepatitis A

Source: Adapted from *Report of the Committee on Infectious Diseases, 1991* (pp 70–72), with permission of the American Academy of Pediatricians, © 1991.

Exclusion criteria must meet:

- the needs of the day care center (criteria must protect other children and staff members and must allow for limitations of staff capabilities)

- the needs of parents (insofar as possible)

PRECAUTIONS IN SPECIAL POPULATIONS

Three groups of children warrant special consideration either because they are unusually susceptible to infection or because they may infect other children. They are children with developmental disabilities, chronic illnesses, or impaired immunity.

Despite the risks of spreading or acquiring infections, children in these special groups require opportunities for socialization. With care and planning, the majority of these children can be safely integrated into day care and school settings. Administrators, teachers, and care providers should work closely with parents and health care providers to establish safe environments for these children, their peers, and staff members who care for them.

Children with Developmental Disabilities

In general, children with developmental disabilities are not particularly susceptible to infection and require no special precautions or procedures. A few categories of disabilities are associated with higher rates of infection, however. Children with spina bifida (meningomyelocele), for example, are particularly prone to urinary tract infections. Although these infections pose no risk to other children or care providers, the staff in day care and preschool settings may be called upon to participate in special preventive procedures, such as intermittent catheterizations of the bladder. Staff should also be alert to signs and symptoms of urinary tract infection, such as fever or foul-smelling urine, and should bring these to the attention of the child's parent (see Chapter 12).

Children with certain disabilities may be especially susceptible to respiratory and ear infections. For example, children with cerebral palsy or neuromuscular conditions may not have an effective cough or may be unable to swallow oral secretions well, which can lead to frequent bouts of pneumonia. Children with Down syndrome seem to have a higher than normal number of respiratory infections, and children with cleft palates have frequent ear infections, which can lead to chronic otitis media with effusion (see Chapter 8). Although these children may have a high incidence of infection, their symptoms are usually no different from those of other children.

Many care providers are concerned that certain infections acquired before or around the time of birth (eg, rubella, CMV, herpes simplex, hepatitis, and AIDS) may persist and be spread to other children or staff members. In some cases these congenital infections pose an unmeasurably small risk to others, and with proper precautions affected children may safely participate in most day care or educational programs. In other cases, special precautions are warranted. (For detailed discussions of these infections and their appropriate management in child care settings, see Chapters 11, 14, and 15.)

Children with Chronic Illnesses

Children with chronic illnesses or prolonged states of debilitation or malnutrition are particularly susceptible to infection. For example, infants with a history of prematurity who have chronic lung disease (bronchopulmonary dysplasia) and children with cystic fibrosis are more likely to have complications of usual respiratory infections. Similarly, children with congenital heart disease may have unusual difficulty with some respiratory viruses. Children with diseases or structural abnormalities of the urinary tract are highly susceptible to infections of the bladder and kidneys. Although it is not always possible to prevent these diseases, care providers should be alert to the symptoms of infections and notify the child's parents and/or physician if they occur. Once treatment is initiated, these children should be able to participate in regular group care activities.

Children with Impaired Immunity

Certain diseases or treatments can lower the body's natural defenses against infection (see Chapter 1). AIDS, cancer, and other chronic diseases of the immune system substantially alter the body's ability to fight infection, allowing even common organisms to become quickly life threatening. In children with previously normal immune systems, some drugs that are used to treat chronic conditions (eg, steroids for nephrotic syndrome) suppress the body's ability to fight infection. Drugs used to prevent rejection of organ transplants or to temper the body's attack on its own organs can also interfere with the normal immune response. In a child with cancer, both the disease itself and the drugs used to treat it inhibit the body's defense mechanisms.

Children with diseases or treatments that affect the immune system may be isolated from other children during periods of particular susceptibility. Their physicians may prescribe special precautions regarding limited exposure to infection, particularly to chickenpox (because this disease can be fatal in individuals with suppressed immunity).

REFERENCES

Adler SP. Cytomegalovirus transmission among children in day care, their mothers and caretakers. *Pediatr Infect Dis J.* 1988; 7:279–285.

American Academy of Pediatrics. *Report of the Committee on Infectious Diseases.* 22nd ed. Elk Grove Village, Ill: American Academy of Pediatrics; 1991.

American Public Health Association, American Academy of Pediatrics. *Caring for Our Children. National Health and Safety Standards: Guidelines for Out-of-Home Child Care Programs.* APHA and AAP, Washington, D.C., and Elk Grove Village, Ill:1992.

Aronson SE, Gilsdorf JR. Prevention and management of infectious diseases in day care. *Pediatr Rev.* 1986; 7:259–268.

Broome CV, Mortimer EA, Katz SL, Fleming DW, Hightower AW. Use of chemoprophylaxis to prevent the spread of Hemophilus influenza B in day-care facilities. *N Engl J Med.* 1987; 316:1226–1228.

Hutto C, Ricks R, Garvie M, Pass RF. Epidemiology of cytomegalovirus infections in young children; day care vs. home care. *Pediatr Infect Dis J.* 1984; 4:149–152.

Kendrick AS, Kaufmann R, Messenger KP (eds). *Healthy Young Children. A Manual for Programs.* Washington, DC: National Association for the Education of Young Children; 1988.

Makintubee S, Istre GR, Ward JI. Transmission of invasive *Haemophilus influenzae* type B disease in day care settings. *J Pediatr.* 1987; 111:180–186.

Murph JR, Bale JF. The natural history of acquired cytomegalovirus infection among children in group day care. *Am J Dis Child.* 1988; 42:843–846.

Murph JR, Bale JF, Murray JC, Stinski MF, and Perlman S. Cytomegalovirus transmission in a midwest day care center: possible relationship to child care practices. *J Pediatr.* 1986; 109:35–39.

Murphy T (guest ed). Infection related to day-care attendance. *Pediatr Ann.* 1991; 20:403–441.

Murphy T, Clements JF, Breedlove JA, Hansen EJ, Seibert GB. Risk of subsequent disease among day-care contacts of patients with systemic *Hemophilus influenzae* type B disease. *N Engl J Med.* 1987; 316:5–10.

Osterholm MT, Reves RR, Murph JR, Pickering LK. Infectious diseases in child day care. *Pediatr Infect Dis J.* 1992; 11:S31–S41.

Pass RF, Hutto SC, Reynolds DW, Polhill RB. Increased frequency of cytomegalovirus infection in children in group day care. *Pediatrics.* 1984; 74:121–126.

Peterson-Sweeney K, Stevens J. Educating child care providers in child health. *Pediatr Nurs.* 1992; 18:37–40.

Wald ER, Guerra N, Byers C. Frequency and severity of infections in day care: three-year follow-up. *J Pediatr.* 1991; 118:509–514.

Chapter 6

Infectious Diseases of Concern for Day Care Providers

Although children are much more likely than adults to acquire infections in the day care setting, a few diseases pose a potential occupational risk for day care providers. This chapter provides information about diseases that pose particular hazards to adults, how they are transmitted, and how they can be prevented.

Day care providers are at risk for acquiring upper respiratory tract infections (colds) and enteric infections with diarrhea. Because these infections are usually mild and self-limited, however, they are not discussed in detail.

DISEASES THAT ARE A RISK PRIMARILY FOR PREGNANT WOMEN

Cytomegalovirus

Cytomegalovirus (CMV), a member of the herpesvirus family of viruses, is commonly transmitted among children in the day care setting (see Chapter 5). The majority of children or adults who become infected have no apparent symptoms of illness. Even so, adults or children whose immune systems are impaired by disease [such as cancer or acquired immunodeficiency syndrome (AIDS)] or medications (such as steroids, drugs used to treat cancer, or drugs used in organ transplant patients) are at risk for severe, overwhelming disease should they become infected with CMV. These individuals may develop severe pneumonia or retinitis, an inflammation of the eye that can result in blindness.

A more frequent concern, however, is the day care provider who may be pregnant or anticipating pregnancy. If a nonimmune woman becomes infected with CMV for the first time during pregnancy, there is a risk that the virus may be transmitted to the fetus, causing birth defects (see Chapter 14). Several recent studies indicate that day care providers and the parents of children in day care are at significantly increased risk for CMV infection compared with the general population (see Table 6-1).

In 1989, a study in Virginia determined that 11% of day care providers employed at day care centers in the Richmond, Virginia, area became infected with CMV each year. This was contrasted with an annual seroconversion (new infection) rate of 2% among female hospital employees in the same geographic area. Women who cared for children younger than 2 years of age were at greatest risk.

A subsequent study performed in Alabama found that 20% of day care workers became infected with CMV each year, a rate that was 10 times higher than expected. In this study, infection was associated with caring for children younger than 3 years for at least 20 hours per week.

A similar study from Iowa found an annual rate of CMV infection of 8% among all day care providers studied. The risk of infection for day care providers varied from center to center, however, and paralleled the risk of infection among children. Providers at centers with higher rates of CMV infection among children had a greater risk of becoming infected. The risk of a provider becoming infected within the following year ranged from 0% at some centers to 22% at one location.

Parents of children in day care are also at increased risk for CMV infection. One study determined that 21% of parents with children in day care became infected during an average of 17 months of observation compared with 0% of parents with children cared for at home (see Table 6-1). Of par-

Table 6-1 Risk of CMV Infection among Day Care Providers and Parents

Population	*Percentage who became infected*
General population	2–5
Day care providers	8–20
Parents with	
No children in day care	0
Children in day care	21
Children in day care and shedding CMV in urine	30
Children in day care younger than 18 months and shedding CMV in urine	45

ents with a child known to be shedding CMV, 30% became infected, and nearly half of parents with a child 18 months of age or younger and shedding CMV became infected. Another study found that 30% of mothers of infected children seroconverted each year compared with 3% of mothers of noninfected children. These studies indicate that the mothers of children in day care are at greatly increased risk for CMV infection.

Recommendations To Prevent the Transmission of Cytomegalovirus to Day Care Providers

CMV is spread by direct contact with body fluids (primarily urine and saliva) that contain the virus.

- Providers should practice good personal hygiene during diaper changes. Disposable gloves can be worn and discarded after each use. Alternatively, careful hand washing with warm, soapy water can be practiced (hand-washing and diapering techniques are described in Appendices B and C).
- Women who anticipate pregnancy may wish to have a blood test to determine whether they have antibodies to CMV. Women who possess antibodies to CMV are immune and generally protected from having a severely affected infant.
- Nonimmune women who are pregnant or anticipating pregnancy may decrease their risk of exposure to CMV by caring only for children older than 3 years.
- Providers should avoid contact with the saliva of children. Avoid kissing children on or around the mouth or on the hands and sharing food, glasses, or eating utensils.
- Children known to be infected with CMV should not be excluded from day care. As many as 50% of all children attending day care may be excreting CMV in their urine or saliva but are undiagnosed. It would be impractical and ineffective to exclude those few children who have been identified.
- Women who are pregnant or anticipating pregnancy should assume that all young children may be shedding CMV and should maintain rigorous personal hygiene and follow universal precautions when contact with any body fluid is likely.

Parvovirus B19

Parvovirus B19 causes erythema infectiosum, also known as fifth disease, in children. This disease is usually mild and is characterized primarily by a distinctive rash giving infected children a "slapped cheek" appearance to their face and a fine, lacy rash on their arms, legs, and trunk, which may disappear and then recur. Although parvovirus causes mild disease in children, adults are at risk for developing painful arthritis. Individuals with certain chronic anemias may have severe worsening of their anemia. Of greatest concern to day care providers, however, is the risk to the fetus if a nonimmune woman becomes infected during pregnancy. During the first half of gestation, parvovirus can cause severe anemia of the fetus, which may ultimately result in heart failure and fetal death. The actual risk of fetal loss after parvovirus infection in the first or second trimester is small, estimated to be 3% to 9%.

Approximately 50% of adults are susceptible (nonimmune) to infection. If exposed to parvovirus by an infected family member, 50% of the susceptible household contacts will become infected. The risk for day care providers or teachers is less than that for family contacts but significantly greater than that for the general population in the community. During a 1988 outbreak of erythema infectiosum in a Connecticut community, 31% of nonimmune day care workers became infected with parvovirus.

Recommendations To Prevent Transmission of Parvovirus B19

Parvovirus is spread from person to person through respiratory secretions.

- Women who are pregnant or expecting to become pregnant can have their immune status determined by a blood test for parvovirus antibody. Those who have antibody can be reassured that they are not at risk for infection even if they are exposed to the virus. In the event of an outbreak of erythema infectiosum, those who are not immune may wish to consider temporary reassignment to non–child care positions. Routine reassignment of pregnant child care workers with unknown immune status is not recommended because 50% or more of these women will be immune. Also, during an outbreak of erythema infectiosum these women will be exposed to the virus in the community as well as at work.
- Careful attention to personal hygiene is important, especially hand washing after wiping a child's nose or face or otherwise coming into contact with saliva or nasal secretions.
- Providers should dispose of soiled tissues properly in a closed, plastic, lined container and should clean contaminated toys, tables, or other surfaces with a bleach–water solution.

- Providers should not kiss children on or around the mouth; share food, eating utensils, or drinking glasses; or allow children to put their hands or other saliva-contaminated objects into the mouth of the child care provider.
- Children with erythema infectiosum need not be excluded from school or day care because they are unlikely to be infectious after the rash is present.

Rubella

The rubella virus causes a mild illness associated with a measleslike rash and enlarged lymph nodes in the neck and at the back of the head (see Chapter 13). The major concern with rubella is the risk to nonimmune pregnant women. If a woman becomes infected with rubella for the first time during the first trimester of pregnancy, there is considerable risk that the virus will be transmitted to the fetus, causing serious birth defects (congenital rubella syndrome; see Chapter 14 for more information).

The last major epidemic of rubella in the United States occurred in the 1960s. Recent studies show, however, that 10% to 20% of young adults are now susceptible to infection. There has also been an alarming increase in the incidence of rubella in this country. In 1988 there were only 225 cases of rubella reported. In 1990 that figure had risen to more than 1,000 cases with 10 confirmed cases of congenital rubella syndrome.

Recommendations To Prevent Transmission of Rubella

Rubella is transmitted by the respiratory route.

- If day care providers are unsure of their immune status, a blood test can determine their immunity. Nonimmune workers who are not pregnant should be immunized with the measles, mumps, and rubella (MMR) vaccine. Those who have antibody against rubella are protected from infection.
- Recommendations for hygienic measures to interrupt transmission of diseases spread by the respiratory route should be followed (see recommendations for prevention of parvovirus infection, above).

Chickenpox (Varicella)

Chickenpox is usually a mild febrile illness with a distinctive, blistering rash in young children (see Chapter 13). In adolescents and adults, however, this virus often produces more serious disease with complications such as pneumonia. For this reason, adults with chickenpox are usually treated with an antiviral drug to minimize the severity of the disease. Pregnant, nonimmune women who become infected with the varicella virus are at even greater risk for serious complications than other adults, especially late in pregnancy. In addition, infection early in gestation can occasionally produce serious birth defects in the fetus (see Chapter 14).

Recommendations To Prevent Transmission of Chickenpox

Chickenpox is transmitted by the respiratory route and also by direct contact with the characteristic skin lesions.

- If a day care worker has never had chickenpox or is unsure about whether he or she has had this virus, a blood test should be performed to determine the provider's immune status. A vaccine to prevent varicella will soon be available for use in normal children and adults. Non-immune day care providers should contact their physician for further information. If a nonimmune pregnant woman is exposed to chickenpox, a special preventive measure (varicella zoster immune globulin) may be recommended. Some previously immune individuals who are taking medication that suppresses their immune system may also be susceptible to infection. These individuals should contact their physician for recommendations.
- Children with chickenpox should be excluded from day care until 6 days after the onset of the rash or until all the lesions have dried and crusted, if this occurs sooner.

OTHER INFECTIONS

Hepatitis A

This virus is commonly transmitted among children attending day care centers. The majority of infected children have mild disease or infection without symptoms and rarely develop jaundice (yellow skin color). Most adults will become noticeably jaundiced, however, and many will become quite ill.

Recommendations To Prevent Transmission of Hepatitis A

Hepatitis A is spread by the fecal-oral route.

- Careful hygiene, particularly with respect to hand washing after diaper changes, before eating or preparing food, or whenever there has been contact with stool, is important (see Guidelines for Preventing Disease Spread in Day Care Centers in Chapter 5).

- If a case of hepatitis A occurs in a child or staff member of a day care center, the local health department will recommend immune globulin for contacts to prevent transmission (see Chapters 5 and 11).

Hepatitis B

Hepatitis B virus causes a serious disease with inflammation of the liver. This disease is rarely transmitted in the day care setting. To date, there have been only a few case reports of day care–related transmission.

Recommendations To Prevent Transmission of Hepatitis B

Hepatitis B is transmitted by direct contact with blood or blood-containing body fluids. It is also transmitted sexually.

- Universal precautions should be used whenever a day care provider anticipates contact with blood or blood-containing body fluids. These precautions are described in detail in Chapter 5 (Guidelines for Preventing Disease Spread in Day Care Centers).
- To use universal precautions, providers must be prepared. Gloves must be readily accessible for cleaning up spills of body fluids or for assisting with an injury. Personnel supervising playground activities or field trips should carry gloves and gauze pads in a plastic bag to ensure their availability in the event of an injury.
- Careful environmental decontamination after blood spills is important (see Chapter 5).
- Recommendations regarding chronic hepatitis B carrier children are discussed in Chapter 5. Remember, there are already chronic hepatitis B carriers attending day care centers. Some of these children are undiagnosed and therefore have not been identified to the day care provider. Therefore, assume that any child in your care may be infected with the hepatitis B virus, and use careful personal and environmental hygiene when dealing with any body fluid.

IMMUNIZATIONS: NOT FOR CHILDREN ONLY

As part of preemployment health screening, all day care providers should have their immunization status assessed (see Table 6-2 for recommendations for healthy adults). Just as for children, child care workers should maintain an updated immunization card. In addition to immunization, day care providers should be screened for tuberculosis during preemployment health assessment. Tuberculosis testing should be repeated at intervals determined by the local health department.

Tetanus and Diphtheria

Tetanus and diphtheria toxoid (Td) must be readministered every 10 years. In the event of certain injuries (see Table 6-3), a physician may recommend reimmunization sooner. More frequent immunization is not recommended because of the risk of increased side effects.

Pertussis

At this time, routine immunization of adults against pertussis is not recommended. As effective, safer vaccines become available, these recommendations may change.

Polio

Immunization of adults in the United States who were not immunized as children is not routinely recommended because of the lack of wild poliovirus in this country. There is a small risk, however, that these unimmunized adults could develop oral poliovirus vaccine–associated poliomyelitis when exposed to the live vaccine virus excreted in the stools of recently immunized children. Unimmunized child care providers may be at particular risk because of the frequent contact with many recently immunized children in diapers and should be immunized with the inactivated poliovirus vaccine.

Table 6-2 Recommendations for Routine Immunization of Adults

Vaccine	*Population*	*Frequency*
Td	All adults	Every 10 years
MMR	All adults*	One dose
Influenza	Adults > 65 years†	Annually
Pneumococcal	Adults > 65 years†	One dose

* In accordance with the Immunization Practices Advisory Committee recommendations for routine immunization (live-virus vaccines are contraindicated in certain persons).

† Also recommended for certain high-risk groups (see Chapter 3 on individual vaccines).

Table 6-3 Recommendations for Tetanus Prevention after Injury

Tetanus immunization status	*Clean minor wound*		*All other wounds**	
	Td	*TIG*	*Td*	*TIG*
Uncertain or < three doses	Yes	No	Yes	Yes
> three doses[†]	No[‡]	No	No[§]	No

TIG—tetanus immune globulin

* For example, wounds contaminated with dirt, saliva, or feces; puncture wounds; frostbite; crush injuries.

† If only three doses of toxoid have been received, a fourth dose of toxoid should be given.

‡ Yes if >10 years since last dose.

§ Yes if > 5 years since last dose.

Source: Adapted from Update on Adult Immunization: Recommendations of the Immunization Practices Advisory Committee, *MMWR* (1991; 40: No. RR-12), November 15, 1991, Centers for Disease Control.

Most adults have been fully immunized as children with the oral poliovirus vaccine. If you have not been immunized or if your immunization status is unknown, contact your physician. In most cases, unimmunized adults should be immunized with the enhanced-potency inactivated poliovirus vaccine (see Chapter 3).

Measles, Mumps, and Rubella

Child care workers may be at increased risk for exposure to these vaccine-preventable childhood illnesses. Adults born after 1956 without either documentation of MMR vaccination after 12 months of age or laboratory documentation of immunity should be immunized with the MMR vaccine. Individuals born before 1957 are generally considered immune to measles because of the epidemic occurrence of measles at that time. In general, MMR is the preferred vaccine for individuals susceptible to measles, mumps, or rubella.

Hemophilus influenzae Type b

Most adults are immune and therefore not at risk for serious *Hemophilus influenzae* type b disease. Individuals with impaired immunity (due to AIDS or other immunodeficiency diseases, sickle cell disease, splenectomy, Hodgkin's disease, or immune suppression secondary to medication) may be at increased risk for disease caused by this bacterium, however. These individuals may benefit from immunization. Providers should consult their physicians for more information and recommendations.

Hepatitis B

Day care transmission of hepatitis B is rare. In 1992, however, the Centers for Disease Control recommended universal immunization against hepatitis B with the three-dose immunization series initiated in the newborn period. It is hoped that eventually the entire American population will be immunized. At this time, hepatitis B vaccination can be offered safely to anyone desiring to be protected. It is particularly important for individuals in high-risk groups (homosexual males, intravenous drug users, heterosexuals with multiple sexual partners, workers in health-related fields, and household contacts of chronic hepatitis B carriers).

The July 1992 standards for employers set by the Occupational Safety and Health Administration dictate that all employees who are expected to have occupational exposure to blood or other potentially infectious material should be offered hepatitis B vaccination. This may apply to the day care center director or other specifically designated person who would routinely be involved in providing first aid. The standards also indicate that personnel who are unvaccinated and who administer first aid in a situation where blood or other potentially infectious material is present should be offered hepatitis B vaccination within 24 hours of the incident. Because it is likely that these regulations will change from time to time, consult your local health department for the latest recommendations.

Influenza

Influenza causes major outbreaks or epidemics of disease each winter. Adults who are at risk for more serious disease or complications should receive the vaccine each fall. Individuals considered at high risk include persons older than 65 years and those with chronic lung or heart disorders (such as asthma or emphysema), chronic metabolic disease (such as diabetes mellitus), kidney disease, certain blood disorders, or altered immune function (including immune suppression caused by medication). In addition, individuals who provide care for children who are in a high-risk category can transmit influenza to these persons and should be vaccinated. The influenza vaccine is safe and can be offered to any person wishing to reduce his or her risk of acquiring influenza.

Pneumococcal Disease

Individuals older than 65 years and those with certain chronic conditions (chronic heart and lung disease, diabetes mellitus, alcoholism, sickle cell disease, absent or poorly functioning spleen, kidney failure, Hodgkin's disease, AIDS, etc) are at risk for severe pneumococcal disease and should be immunized.

REFERENCES

Bale JF, Murph JR. The risk of cytomegalovirus infection in hospital personnel and child care providers: a review. *Pediatr Rev Commun*. 1991; 4:233–246.

Centers for Disease Control. Hepatitis B virus: a comprehensive strategy for eliminating transmission in the United States through universal childhood vaccination. Recommendations of the Immunization Practices Advisory Committee (ACIP). *MMWR*. 1991; 40.

Centers for Disease Control. Rubella prevention. Recommendations of the Immunization Practices Advisory Committee (ACIP). *MMWR*. 1990; 39.

Dobbins JG, Adler SP, Pass RF, Bale JF, Grillner L, Stewart JA. Risks and benefits of cytomegalovirus transmission in child day care. *Pediatr Rev Commun*. In press.

Murph JR, Baron JC, Brown CK, Ebelhack CL, Bale JF. The occupational risk of cytomegalovirus infection among day-care providers. *JAMA*. 1991; 265:603-608.

US Department of Labor. *First Aid Providers May Receive Hepatitis B Vaccine upon Exposure, OSHA Says* (news release). Washington DC: Office of Information, US Department of Labor; 1992.

US Department of Labor. *Occupational Exposure to Bloodborne Pathogens*. Washington DC: Occupational Safety and Health Administration; 1992.

Part II

Specific Infections of Children

Chapter 7

Diseases of the Eyes and Mouth

DISEASES OF THE EYES

Blepharitis

Blepharitis is an inflammation of the eyelid margins that is characterized by irritation, burning, or itching. This condition can be caused by the bacterium *Staphylococcus aureus*, or it can accompany seborrhea, a chronic inflammatory disease characterized by greasy scaling and crusting of the eyelids, scalp (cradle cap), eyebrows, face, diaper area, and other areas of the body. Treatment for both types of blepharitis is daily cleansing with a moistened cotton applicator to remove scales. If the blepharitis is bacterial, an antibiotic ointment is also applied to the lid margins.

Stye

A stye (hordeolum) is an infection of the lash follicle or sweat glands of the eyelid, usually with the bacterium *Staphylococcus aureus*. The eyelid is red and swollen, and an abscess forms within the eyelid along or near the lid margin. A stye is treated with warm compresses and, in some cases, topical antibiotics. At times, the abscess must be drained by a physician. Some children are prone to recurrent styes.

Nasolacrimal (Tear) Duct Obstruction

Blocked tear ducts are a relatively common problem of infancy. They cause excessive tearing, which is usually apparent within the first few weeks after birth, and recurrent eye infection or conjunctivitis. Tears, which would normally drain through the nasolacrimal duct into the nose, cannot do so because of an obstruction of the duct. Of all blocked tear ducts, 80% to 90% will open spontaneously within the first 9 months of life. Until the obstruction is opened (either spontaneously or through probing by an ophthalmologist), these children are prone to recurrent infection. These infections are usually mild and respond well to antibiotic drops or ointment applied to the eye. In addition, massaging the area over the duct may hasten resolution. Occasionally, nasolacrimal duct obstruction may result in a more serious condition called dacryocystitis.

Dacryocystitis

Dacryocystitis is an infection of the lacrimal sac of the tear duct that occurs in infants who have nasolacrimal duct obstruction. This problem is characterized by redness and swelling over the lacrimal sac (located at the inner corner of the eye). Infants with dacryocystitis may appear quite ill and always require systemic antibiotics (by mouth or intravenously). If this condition is suspected, a physician should be consulted.

Conjunctivitis

The conjunctivae, the clear membranes lining the inside of the lid and the white part of the eyes, can react to a wide range of bacterial and viral agents, allergens (grass, ragweed), irritants (dust, smoke), toxins (gaseous fumes, cleaning agents), and generalized body illnesses (measles, Kawasaki disease). The linings of the eyes and lids become mildly to fiery red. There may be excessive tearing and a discharge of pus, especially if the conjunctivitis is infectious (usually called pinkeye).

The most common infectious causes of conjunctivitis are viruses and bacteria such as staphylococci, streptococci, pneumococci, and *Hemophilus influenzae*. Antibiotic drops are commonly instilled if bacterial conjunctivitis is suspected. There is no specific treatment for most types of viral conjunctivitis.

Redness of the eye, particularly in a young child, should be evaluated by a health care provider to determine the cause and extent of involvement of the eyes and lids as well as the appropriate treatment. Usually, superficial infections of the eyes are not serious. If nonbacterial, they resolve without treatment; if bacterial, they can be easily treated with drops or ointment. In some cases, however, such as when the conjunctivitis is caused by herpes simplex virus, delay in treatment can cause considerable damage to the eye. Moreover, an infection of the eyelids may signal infection in other parts of the eye, or it can spread to deeper tissues around the eye, causing periorbital cellulitis, a particularly serious condition that may require hospitalization and intravenous antibiotics.

Infectious types of conjunctivitis are contagious. Caretakers should wash their hands well after contact with affected children. Towels and other objects used by an affected child should not be shared with others until the infection has cleared. The child should be isolated or kept at home until the eye drainage ceases.

DISEASES OF THE MOUTH

Thrush

Thrush (oral moniliasis or candidiasis) is a fungal infection of the mouth characterized by white, flaky patches on the inside of the cheek and on the gums and tongue (see Color Plate 1). This condition is more common in newborn infants, although it may continue to occur periodically throughout infancy.

Thrush is caused by *Candida albicans*, a regular inhabitant of the skin, mouth, intestine, and vagina. Normally, this yeast does not cause problems because other microorganisms keep it in check. If the balance is upset, however, say by administration of an antibiotic (eg, amoxicillin to treat an ear infection), the fungus can proliferate and cause recognizable thrush. Thrush can also be a sign of abnormalities of the body's immune system, which is why children with persistent infections are sometimes evaluated for signs of underlying disease.

The oral lesions may be confused with milk, which temporarily adheres to the same places, especially inside the cheeks. Most experienced clinicians readily recognize thrush, however, and treat it without any special tests (although the diagnosis can be confirmed by direct microscopic examination and culture of scrapings from lesions).

To treat thrush, an antifungal solution is placed in the mouth. The amount and timing of administration should be directed by a physician. Some infants with thrush have accompanying monilial diaper rash (see Chapters 13 and 16), which is treated with a topical ointment.

Herpes Simplex Infections

The herpes simplex virus is ubiquitous and causes infections at any time during the year. This virus can cause serious illness in infants younger than 28 days (see Chapter 14). In other children, however, the most commonly recognized sign of infection is oral lesions. These are usually caused by type 1 herpes simplex virus. A rare manifestation of herpes simplex infection is encephalitis (see Chapter 9).

First exposure to the virus usually results in few or no symptoms. Some children, however, develop a generalized infection of the mouth (acute herpetic gingivostomatitis). Ulcerated sores in or around the mouth appear abruptly or, less commonly, over a period of days, causing pain, salivation, foul-smelling breath, refusal to eat, and high fever. Full recovery requires 1 to 2 weeks. A major problem with gingivostomatitis is persuading the child with a sore mouth to take fluids. In some cases, hospitalization and intravenous fluids are required.

The herpes simplex virus is transmitted from person to person. Most mild oral herpes lesions go unnoticed, and affected children continue in school or day care, potentially infecting others with this common disease. Acute gingivostomatitis, on the other hand, is obvious, and children with this condition are kept at home because of illness as well as communicability.

In some individuals, latent herpes simplex virus can be reactivated by an upper respiratory infection, fever, sunlight, or stress, producing a lesion (also called a cold sore or fever blister) on the lips. Until this lesion is crusted over, the virus is actively shed and can be transmitted from mouth to mouth or from mouth to object to mouth. A young child with an active cold sore should be isolated from other children until the lesion is crusted over, and toys and other objects mouthed by a child with a herpetic lesion should be soaked in a solution of 1 part chlorine bleach to 10 parts water.

Older children and adults with active lesions pose less of a problem, because they are unlikely to transmit the virus directly. Such individuals should avoid mouth-to-mouth contact with others. Caretakers with active (not yet crusted over) herpes lesions should avoid contact with infants younger than 28 days or wear a mask. Proper hand washing by all caretakers is also essential before contact with newborns.

Hand, Foot, and Mouth Disease

Hand, foot, and mouth disease, a syndrome caused by certain enteroviruses, is characterized by a distinctive rash, usually in the mouth and on the soles of the hands and feet, although it can also appear elsewhere on the body (see Color Plate 2, a and b). Although epidemics of this illness may occur, it is generally a mild disease that resolves without treatment.

Herpangina

Herpangina (which, despite the sound of its name, has nothing to do with herpesvirus or pains in the chest) is an acute disorder caused by an enterovirus (coxsackievirus or echovirus). Herpangina is characterized by rash (including small ulcerations) on the soft palate and throat. Other signs and symptoms include a sore throat, manifested by difficulty swallowing and reluctance to eat or drink, and an abrupt elevation in temperature to as high as 105°F (40.6°C). There may also be headache or abdominal pain. The fever lasts from 1 to 4 days, and the sores in the mouth take about 1 week to heal. Treatment consists of medications for pain and fever. Children should be encouraged to take bland, nonacidic fluids. Popsicles or ice chips may be readily accepted.

Canker Sores

Canker sores (aphthous ulcers) are painful ulcerations of the mouth. They usually occur on the inside of the cheek or on the gums but can appear on the tongue or palate as well. The cause of canker sores is uncertain, although some individuals seem to be more susceptible than others. Ulcerations have been attributed to reactions to foods, allergens, and drugs as well as to infections, emotional stress, and injury.

The ulcerations heal in about 1 week; there is no known means of shortening their duration or, for that matter, of preventing them in the first place. Anesthetic mouthwashes may help reduce discomfort in older children. Acidic foods, such as citrus fruits, should be avoided. Canker sores are sometimes confused with herpetic gingivostomatitis (described above).

Mumps

Mumps, a disease caused by a paramyxovirus, is less severe in children than in adults. Each year 1 to 2 persons in every 100,000 acquire this disease. Two thirds of affected persons have puffy cheeks, which are caused by swelling of the salivary glands. Other symptoms include fever, diarrhea, and a generally sick feeling.

Symptoms appear 2 to 3 weeks after the airborne paramyxovirus enters the respiratory tract. Diagnosis is based on the swollen cheeks or the presence of antibodies to the mumps virus. The period of highest communicability is from several days before the onset of salivary gland swelling to 1 week after onset. Infected children should be isolated during this period (at least from the time mumps is recognized), especially from adults who have no history of mumps infection.

There is no specific treatment for mumps, although it can be prevented by a vaccine that is usually administered along with vaccines against measles (rubeola) and German measles (rubella) at 15 months of age.

Possible complications of mumps include inflammation of the coverings of the brain and spinal cord (meningoencephalitis, see Chapter 9), swelling of the testicles in postpubertal males, acute pancreatitis in children, and, rarely, hearing impairment and damage to other tissues such as the kidneys and joints.

Dental Disease

Poor oral hygiene and failure to administer fluoride (either through the water supply or in dietary supplements) set the stage for tooth decay and gum (periodontal) disease. The metabolic action of bacteria on carbohydrates and other substances produces acids and toxins in the plaque. These toxins demineralize tooth enamel, producing cavities, and irritate tissues around the teeth, causing inflammation and swelling of the gums (gingivitis). The gingivitis, unless given proper attention, can eventually progress to the bone around the teeth, resulting in damaged or lost teeth.

Lengthy bottle feedings of milk, juice, or sweetened liquids once teeth have erupted typically cause decay (called nursing caries) of the primary upper front teeth and first primary molars.

Prevention is the best treatment. Teeth should be brushed as soon as they begin to erupt. A convenient method is to place the infant in a cradle formed by two adults sitting knee to knee. One stabilizes and interacts with the child while the other wields a small multitufted soft brush that effectively cleans the teeth and massages the gums. Toothpaste is not necessary in young children. As children grow, they should gradually become more involved in the cleaning process.

Children should be seen by a dentist within 6 months of the first tooth eruption to begin a comprehensive preventive dentistry program that can reduce or eliminate dental disease.

Sore Throats

This topic is discussed in Chapter 10.

REFERENCES

American Academy of Pediatrics. *Report of the Committee on Infectious Diseases.* 22nd ed. Elk Grove Village, Ill: American Academy of Pediatrics; 1991.

Behrman RE, Kliegman RM, eds. *Nelson Textbook of Pediatrics.* 14th ed. Philadelphia, Pa: Saunders; 1992.

Gellis SS, Kagan BM. *Current Pediatric Therapy.* 13th ed. Philadelphia, Pa: Saunders; 1990.

Rudolph AM, Hoffman JIE, eds. *Pediatrics.* 19th ed. Norwalk, Conn: Appleton & Lange; 1991.

Chapter 8

Ear Infections

Otitis media is an inflammation of the middle ear in which the middle ear space becomes filled with fluid. If this fluid contains bacteria and pus, and if the signs and symptoms of middle ear inflammation are of recent onset, the condition is called acute otitis media. If the fluid is clear and without evidence of infection, the condition is called otitis media with effusion (also called secretory or serous otitis media). In contrast, external otitis (swimmer's ear) is an inflammation of the outer ear, ear canal, and outer surface of the eardrum (tympanic membrane).

The ear is composed of three parts: the external ear, which includes the outer ear (helix) and the ear canal as far as the eardrum; the middle ear, an air-filled space behind the eardrum containing the small bony structures (ossicles) that help transmit sound; and the inner ear, which includes nerves and fluid-filled structures that are necessary for hearing and maintaining balance (Figure 8-1). The eustachian tube connects the middle ear with the nasopharynx (the area where the nasal cavity and throat join). This tube has three main purposes: to ventilate the air-filled cavity of the middle ear so that there is equal air pressure on both sides of the eardrum, to drain fluid produced in the middle ear into the nasopharynx, and to protect the middle ear from secretions and other materials in the nasopharynx.

ACUTE OTITIS MEDIA

Acute otitis media is one of the most common illnesses in children. Only mild upper respiratory infections (the common cold) and well-child examinations are more frequent reasons for a visit to a physician. As much as one fourth of a pediatrician's practice may be related solely to the diagno-

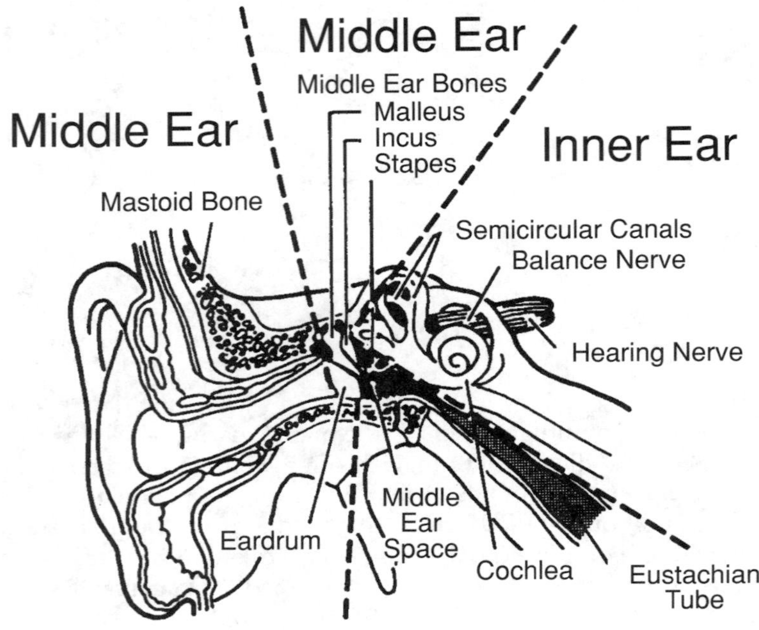

Figure 8-1 The ear

sis and treatment of ear infections, and the annual health care costs of this disease in the United States alone amount to more than $2 billion.

Otitis media occurs most often in children between the ages of 6 and 36 months, but it is also prevalent throughout the preschool years and becomes relatively rare only after age 10 years. Half of all children in this country have at least one episode of acute otitis media before their first birthday, and 10% have three or more such episodes. Two thirds of all children have at least one infection by their third birthday.

The number of reported cases of otitis media has increased over the past 10 years. This increase may reflect such factors as improved diagnostic techniques, resistant strains of bacteria, and increased enrollment in group day care (clustering large groups of children increases the risk for respiratory infections, predisposing these children to otitis media).

Other groups at increased risk for developing acute otitis media include Hispanic and native American children, children with Down syndrome or cleft palate, children living in households with many family members, children whose parents or siblings have a history of recurrent ear infections, and children in group day care. Otitis media is more prevalent among boys, lower socioeconomic groups, and children fed by bottle-propping. The earlier in life the first episode of acute otitis media occurs, the more likely the child is to experience frequent and severe recurrences.

Cause

Eustachian tube dysfunction appears to precipitate episodes of acute otitis media. In young children the eustachian tube is softer and more collapsible than in the adult, and the muscles responsible for periodically opening the tube to allow drainage of secretions may not be completely developed. Frequently, an upper respiratory infection causes inflammation with swelling and increased fluid production in the middle ear, predisposing the child to infection by bacteria.

Acute otitis media is almost always treated as a bacterial infection. Several different bacteria can cause this condition, including *Streptococcus pneumoniae, Hemophilus influenzae, Moraxella catarrhalis,* group A streptococci, and *Staphylococcus aureus.* In the first few weeks of life, acute ear infections can also be caused by group B streptococci, *Chlamydia trachomatis,* or enteric (gastrointestinal) bacteria such as *Klebsiella pneumoniae* and *Escherichia coli.*

Contrary to popular belief, wind does not cause (or worsen) ear infections. Infections of the middle ear are also not caused by swimming or allowing bath water to enter the outer ear.

Signs and Symptoms

Acute otitis media frequently accompanies or follows an upper respiratory infection. Although the signs and symptoms of acute otitis media can be mild or absent, more often the child appears acutely ill.

Young children, particularly infants, may be irritable and restless, wake frequently from sleep, feed poorly, and tug or hit at their ears. Older children with acute otitis media may complain of earache or headache and hearing impairment. In rare cases, balance may be impaired. Ear infections can be accompanied by diarrhea, a green or yellow nasal discharge, and at times an eye infection (conjunctivitis, pinkeye). If the eardrum ruptures, there may be a foul-smelling drainage that contains pus or blood. Because this drainage releases the pressure behind the eardrum (the major source of pain), a child who has been crying inconsolably may subsequently become quiet and appear to be much more comfortable.

Children with uncomplicated acute otitis media often do not have a fever. In fact, a high fever usually prompts a physician to look for a complication of this condition or some other problem.

Diagnosis

Children with symptoms of otitis media are examined with a pneumatic otoscope. This instrument allows the physician to view the eardrum and to assess its mobility by creating positive and negative pressure within the ear canal (Figure 8-2).

Normally, the eardrum is pinkish-gray and translucent with distinct bony landmarks (Figure 8-3), and it moves freely when pressure is applied through the otoscope. During an infection, however, the eardrum appears red, white, or yellow and is opaque and lusterless, and it lacks the normal landmarks. The eardrum is immobile or slow to respond to pressure, and it may bulge into the ear canal because of fluid within the middle ear space.

Management

Before antibiotics were routinely used to treat acute otitis media, most children either recovered spontaneously (often after rupture of the eardrum) or had their eardrums surgically opened to allow the pus to drain (a

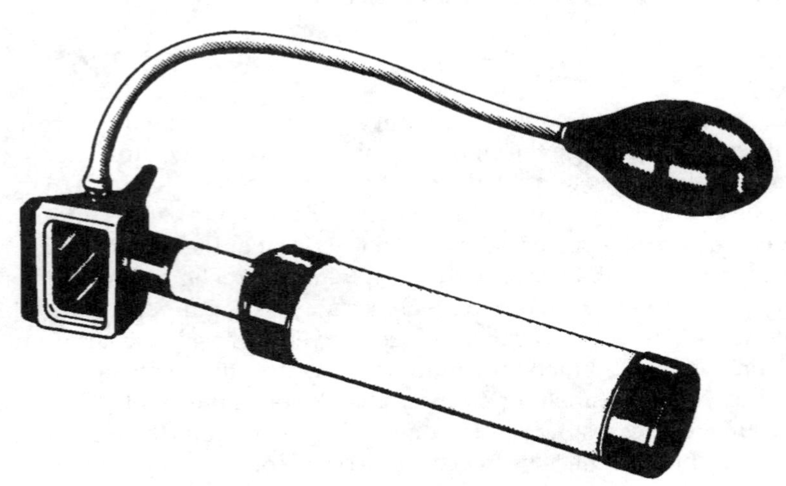

Figure 8-2 Otoscope

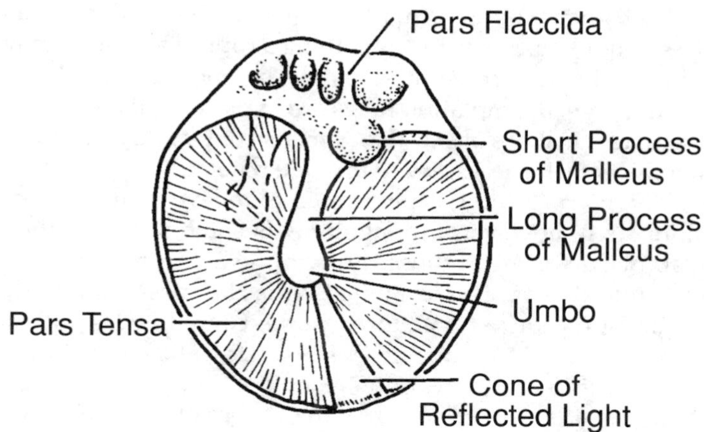

Figure 8-3 The eardrum

procedure known as a myringotomy). Today, although spontaneous recovery may occur, antibiotics are given to all children with acute otitis media to shorten the duration of the illness and to prevent complications, such as chronic ear drainage and mastoiditis (a serious infection of the air cells located behind the ear). A number of antibiotics are effective in the treatment of ear infections. Selection is based on safety, efficacy, expense, and frequency of administration.

Normally, antibiotic therapy of acute otitis media results in significant improvement within 48 hours. The child is less irritable and feverish and is eating and sleeping better. When this does not happen, or if the symptoms worsen at any time, the child should be reevaluated by a physician to determine whether the problem is an ineffective antibiotic, failure to take the prescribed dosage (noncompliance), or development of a complicating condition (eg, pneumonia, bacteremia, or mastoiditis). If the reason for lack of improvement is antibiotic failure, a second (and in rare cases a third) antibiotic may be prescribed.

Because in most instances acute ear infections respond rapidly to appropriate antibiotic treatment, it is not usually necessary to identify the infecting organism. Exceptions may include infants younger than 6 weeks, children with malignancy or a compromised immune system, children who have extreme ear pain or who appear seriously ill, some treatment failures, and children who develop a complication (eg, mastoiditis). In these cases, samples of the infecting organism may be obtained by inserting a needle through the eardrum and removing pus, a procedure known as tympanocentesis.

Pain caused by acute otitis media should be treated with an analgesic, such as acetaminophen. Eardrops containing a topical analgesic may help relieve pain. Eardrops such as these, however, should never be used if there is ear drainage, if ventilation tubes are in place, or if a ruptured eardrum is suspected. In cases of extreme pain, one or two doses of codeine at 4-hour intervals may be necessary to provide relief.

Occasionally, myringotomy is performed to relieve pain and speed recovery. More often, however, myringotomy is combined with the insertion of small plastic or metal tubes through the eardrum that drain and ventilate the middle ear. This combination is the most commonly performed surgical procedure for children in the United States and is used most often to prevent recurrent episodes of acute otitis media in children prone to this condition or to treat otitis media with effusion that persists for more than 3 or 4 months. The insertion of tubes often requires general anesthesia but can usually be performed on an outpatient basis. Because the tubes usually fall out in 6 to 9 months, they must be inserted a second time in approximately 20% of cases.

Although ventilation tubes are often beneficial, they occasionally cause complications such as chronic ear drainage, persistent perforation at the site of tube insertion, scarring and thinning of the eardrum, and formation of a growth (cholesteatoma) in the middle ear. Before considering ventilation tubes, many physicians—including ear, nose, and throat specialists—try to prevent recurrences of acute otitis media with low daily doses of an antibiotic (prophylactic antibiotic therapy), particularly during the winter months, when the incidence of otitis media is highest. Several antibiotics have been proven safe and effective in preventing this disease. Two of the most commonly used are amoxicillin and sulfisoxazole.

To date, there is no evidence that decongestants with or without antihistamines are useful in preventing or treating otitis media during an upper respiratory infection. Moreover, these medications cause some children to develop behavior disturbances (such as drowsiness or hyperactivity), which may be worse than the discomfort of a stuffy nose.

Complications

The most frequently seen complications of otitis media are hearing loss, perforation of the eardrum, scarring of the eardrum (tympanosclerosis), and chronic otitis media with effusion.

Hearing Loss

The most prevalent complication of otitis media is hearing loss, which is usually conductive. Conductive deafness is generally a mild, correctable type of hearing loss. It is caused most often by fluid in the middle ear, although conditions unrelated to otitis media such as accumulated wax or structural problems (eg, incomplete formation) of the ear canal can also impede sound conduction.

Conductive hearing loss can be persistent or fluctuating and is usually reversible. Permanent loss can occur, however, as a result of tympanosclerosis, excessive growth of fibrous tissue within the middle ear (adhesive otitis), or disruption of the middle ear bones (ossicular discontinuity). When infection, on rare occasions, spreads into the inner ear, irreversible sensorineural hearing loss (nerve deafness) can also occur.

Perforation of the Eardrum

Perforation (rupture) of the eardrum is usually a result of an acute infection, although it can also occur with chronic otitis media with effusion. A small perforation is usually of no consequence and heals spontaneously. Large perforations, on the other hand, may result in significant conductive hearing loss. Some require surgical closure.

Eardrum Scarring

Eardrum scarring (tympanosclerosis) can be caused by chronic or recurrent middle ear disease or trauma due to ventilation tubes.

Cholesteatoma

Cholesteatoma, a growth in the middle ear composed of old skin and debris, can occur in the middle ear as a result of chronic middle ear inflammation or the presence of ventilation tubes. Surgical removal is necessary to prevent further growth of the mass, which can erode vital structures in the ear, most commonly the middle ear ossicles.

Mastoiditis

Mastoiditis is a serious infection of the mastoid air cells behind the ear. Treatment consists of tympanocentesis or myringotomy and intravenous antibiotics. Occasionally, more extensive surgical intervention is required to prevent spread of the infection. The widespread use of antibiotics for acute otitis media has made this complication a rare occurrence.

Labyrinthitis

Labyrinthitis occurs when inflammation or infection extends into the inner ear. Before antibiotics, bacterial labyrinthitis sometimes accompanied acute otitis media. Today, serous labyrinthitis, the accumulation of clear fluid in and around the semicircular canals, is more common. Because balance is a function of the semicircular canal, the child with labyrinthitis may complain of dizziness and have frequent falls. Other symptoms of this condition include nausea, vomiting, hearing loss, ringing in the ears, and rapid, jerky involuntary eye movements (nystagmus).

Systemic Complications

In addition to complications within the ear itself, acute otitis media is occasionally accompanied or followed by serious systemic complications such as pneumonia, bacterial infection of the blood stream (bacteremia), and meningitis. For this reason, otitis media should never be diagnosed or antibiotics prescribed on the basis of a phone call alone. Whenever an ear infection is suspected, the child should be seen by a physician in an office setting where a complete medical history can be taken, a physical examination can be performed, and therapy can be recommended. Likewise, the child who does not appear to be responding to appropriate antibiotic therapy should be reevaluated by a physician before a change in treatment is made.

Learning Impairment

Children with long-term moderate or severe hearing loss may experience at least temporary language delay and learning impairment. Children with brief or fluctuating hearing losses, which are often seen with recurrent episodes of acute or serous otitis media, may also have problems with language development. This can be particularly significant for children with other developmental impairments.

Adverse Reactions to Antibiotic Therapy

Complications can arise as a result of antibiotic therapy. Diarrhea and yeast infections of the mouth and diaper area occur frequently. Skin rashes are also relatively common. Certain rashes, however, particularly those with red, raised welts (hives), may signify an allergic reaction to the antibiotic.

Recommendations

Children with symptoms of an ear infection should be seen by a physician for an accurate diagnosis. An otoscopic examination of the ears is an important part of the physician's evaluation of any ill child.

Children being treated for acute otitis media should receive medication according to the schedule prescribed by the physician, although it is not usually necessary to wake a sleeping child to give an antibiotic. Most antibiotics can be given without regard to meals. Antibiotics are usually prescribed for 10 to 14 days. The entire course of medication should be given, even if the child appears to be back to normal in 2 or 3 days. Stopping the antibiotic prematurely can result in a recurrence of the infection.

Significant improvement of acute otitis media should occur within 48 hours after treatment is begun. At times, however, the treatment may fail or a complication may develop. Parents should be notified and the child reevaluated by a physician if any of the following symptoms occur:

- fever persisting more than 48 hours after antibiotic therapy has begun or fever that begins during the course of antibiotic therapy
- severe, persistent earache
- persistent fussiness and irritability, a poor appetite, or frequent awakening from naps or at night after the second day of antibiotic treatment
- extreme lethargy or irritability at any time
- severe, persistent headache or stiff neck
- inability to be comforted
- failure to respond to and interact with the environment and significant adults
- blurred or double vision and difficulty with balance
- seizures
- other signs of worsening

Antibiotics that have been prescribed to prevent ear infections are usually administered daily. Antibiotic prophylaxis that is begun after symptoms of a cold are well established may not be as effective in preventing ear infections.

Common side effects of antibiotics include diarrhea, nausea, vomiting, abdominal pain and cramping, skin rashes, and yeast infections of the mouth or diaper area. If any of these symptoms are persistent or severe, a physician should be consulted. Occasionally, antibiotics cause serious allergic reactions. Any of the following signs and symptoms should be reported to a physician immediately:

- an itchy, hive-like rash
- swelling (edema) of any part of the body but particularly of the face, neck, or throat (swelling of the throat can make breathing difficult)
- difficulty breathing due to spasms of the small airways (an asthma-like attack with wheezing)

- shock, manifested by cold, clammy skin, dizziness or lightheadedness, and low blood pressure

Acute ear infections are not considered contagious, and affected children need not be excluded from school or child care if they are feeling well enough to participate in normal activities.

Generally speaking, children with a perforated eardrum or tubes should not swim or participate in other activities that would permit water or debris to enter the ears. Some tubes are designed to allow swimming or water play, however, and other children may have devices that fit in the ear canal to prevent water entry. Children with otitis media who have an intact eardrum need not be restricted from swimming.

An important part of any therapy is follow-up evaluation by the child's physician at appropriate intervals. All children with acute otitis media should be seen within 2 weeks after treatment is begun.

OTITIS MEDIA WITH EFFUSION

This condition has various synonyms, including serous, secretory, and nonsuppurative otitis media. Children with otitis media with effusion are usually asymptomatic. The middle ear is filled with fluid, but there are no signs or symptoms of acute infection.

Cause

Fluid accumulates in the middle ear whenever eustachian tube dysfunction occurs. It is possible that for some children otitis media with effusion occurs intermittently, and for brief periods of time, throughout childhood. Middle ear fluid commonly persists for weeks to months after an episode of acute otitis media. After their first ear infection, 70% of children have fluid remaining in the middle ear after 2 weeks of antibiotic treatment. This fluid persists for 1 month in 40% of children and for 2 months in 20%.

Signs and Symptoms

In children with otitis media with effusion, the eardrum is sluggish or immobile but without evidence of inflammation. Usually there are no symptoms, although hearing loss or intermittent pain can occur.

Diagnosis

Like acute otitis media, otitis media with effusion can be detected with an otoscope. Another diagnostic instrument for detecting middle ear fluid is the impedance tympanometer. Commonly used by physicians, audiologists, and staff in school screening programs, tympanometry provides an objective measure of eardrum mobility. Use of this instrument is safe, painless, and accurate in children older than 7 months. A rubber plug seals the ear canal, and then a fixed-frequency tone sounds while a pump varies the air pressure within the ear canal. A microphone measures changes in the sound reflected from the surface of the eardrum as it moves (or fails to move) at different pressure levels (Figure 8-4).

Movement of the eardrum is displayed graphically on a record called a tympanogram. Typical tympanogram patterns are shown in Figure 8-5. Type A is a normal pattern, showing normal eardrum movement and atmospheric pressure in the middle ear. Type B is abnormal, showing reduced eardrum movement. Fluid has displaced some or all of the air that is normally present in the middle ear space. This pattern is consistently associated with middle ear fluid. Type C is also abnormal. Although eardrum movement may be normal, middle ear pressure is negative. This pattern is sometimes associated with middle ear fluid.

Management

Treatment for otitis media with effusion is less well defined than that for acute otitis media. Acceptable approaches include watchful waiting (be-

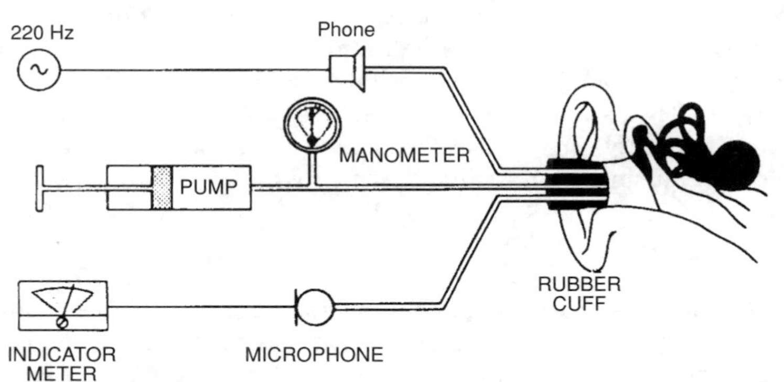

Figure 8-4 Schematic diagram of the impedance tympanometer. *Source*: Reprinted with permission from *Pediatrics* (1976; 58:199), Copyright © 1976, American Academy of Pediatrics.

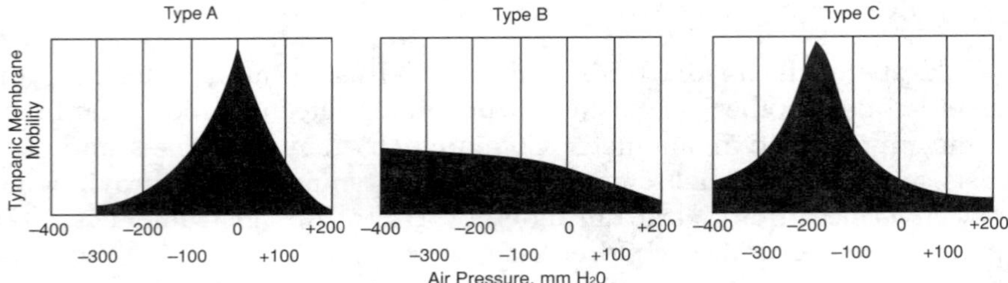

Figure 8-5 Typical tympanogram patterns

cause the majority of cases clear spontaneously), administering prophylactic antibiotics to prevent reinfection in the otitis-prone child, a complete course of antibiotic treatment at full therapeutic doses (because some effusions, even without frank inflammation, contain bacteria), and placement of ventilation tubes if the effusion fails to resolve in 3 to 4 months.

Children receiving antibiotic prophylaxis for otitis media with effusion should be evaluated at 6- to 8-week intervals for resolution or persistence of fluid. Children with ventilation tubes should be monitored at 8- to 12-week intervals for sloughing of the tubes or complications.

Complications

Otitis media with effusion can cause many of the same complications as acute otitis media, including hearing loss (with potential adverse effects on cognitive and language development), perforation, tympanosclerosis, and cholesteatoma. Chronic inflammation can also result in adhesive otitis, which is characterized by a proliferation of fibrous tissue within the middle ear. The ossicles can become embedded in this tissue, resulting in impaired mobility, or they can become eroded and discontinuous from each other, causing a conductive hearing loss.

Recommendations

As a part of the routine well-child examination, all children should receive a pneumatic otoscopic examination and a brief assessment of language acquisition skills. After an episode of acute otitis media or otitis media with effusion, the child should be examined periodically to ensure that the fluid has resolved, that the middle ear has returned to normal, and that no complications have developed.

EXTERNAL OTITIS

External otitis is, as mentioned earlier, an inflammation of the outer ear, ear canal, and outer surface of the eardrum.

Cause

External otitis can be caused by various bacteria, notably *Pseudomonas aeruginosa*, and fungi that thrive in warm, moist environments.

Symptoms and Diagnosis

A child with external otitis often complains of pain and itching, which may be severe. The ear canal is red, swollen, and tender with a cheesy discharge. Pulling the outer ear may produce extreme pain (uncomplicated acute otitis media, by contrast, usually does not cause pain when the outer ear is pulled).

Management

Cleansing and removing debris from the ear canal is the most important part of therapy. A cotton wisp is saturated with an antibiotic preparation. The cotton is inserted deep into the ear canal, where it acts as a wick to cleanse the canal and eliminate bacteria. This cotton wick is changed three or four times during waking hours. If the infection does not respond to cleansing measures and topical antibiotics, cultures should be obtained for fungi and bacteria and appropriate treatment initiated.

External otitis usually does not require systemic antibiotic therapy (taken by mouth or injection). When acute otitis media (which occasionally accompanies external otitis) or mastoiditis is suspected, however, systemic antibiotics may be used along with antibiotic eardrops and cleansing measures.

Recommendations

Swimmers prone to recurrent episodes of external otitis should limit the amount of time they spend in the water, dry their ears thoroughly after swimming, and use an acetic acid preparation (available at any pharmacy) after each day's swimming. Some children may also need to use the acetic acid solution in the morning and at bedtime to prevent recurrences.

REFERENCES

Bluestone CD. Current management of chronic suppurative otitis media in infants and children. *Pediatr Infect Dis J*. 1989; 7:S137–S140.

Bluestone CD. Management of otitis media in infants and children: current role of old and new antimicrobial agents. *Pediatr Infect Dis J*. 1988; 7:S129–S136.

Bluestone CD, Klein JO, eds. *Otitis Media in Infants and Children*. Philadelphia, Pa: Saunders, 1988.

Giebink GS. Progress in understanding the pathophysiology of otitis media. *Pediatr Rev*. 1989; 11:133–138.

McCracken GH. Management of acute otitis media with effusion. *Pediatr Infect Dis J*. 1988; 7:442–445.

Paradise JL. On tympanostomy tubes: rationale, results, reservations, and recommendations. *Pediatrics*. 1977; 60:86–90.

Paradise JL. Otitis media in infants and children. *Pediatrics*. 1980; 65:917–943.

Paradise JL, Smith CG, Bluestone CD. Tympanometric detection of middle ear effusion in infants and young children. *Pediatrics*. 1976; 58:198–210.

Teele DW, Klein JO, Rosner B, and the Greater Boston Otitis Media Study Group. Epidemiology of otitis media during the first seven years of life in children in greater Boston: a prospective, cohort study. *J Infect Dis*. 1989; 160:83–94.

Chapter 9

Meningitis, Encephalitis, and Other Infections of the Nervous System

MENINGITIS

Meningitis is an infection or inflammation of the leptomeninges, the membranes that cover the brain and spinal cord. If meningitis is caused by a virus, the illness is usually brief and benign, posing little or no threat to most healthy children or adults. By contrast, meningitis caused by bacteria can be life threatening. Before the availability of the vaccine for *Hemophilus influenzae* type b (once the most common bacterial cause of meningitis in young children), meningitis affected at least 1 child in every 400 younger than 5 years.

Cause

Meningitis can be caused by many different microorganisms, including viruses, bacteria, and, less commonly, fungi or parasites. A meningitis caused by factors other than bacteria is often referred to as an aseptic meningitis. Although many different viral agents can be associated with meningitis in children (see Table 9-1), echoviruses and coxsackieviruses (collectively called the nonpolio enteroviruses) account for a large proportion of cases. They are distributed worldwide and spread from person to person, usually through contact with the saliva or feces of infected individuals. Infections with these viruses are seasonal, occurring in the summer and fall.

Bacterial meningitis, which poses a far more serious threat to children than viral meningitis, can be caused by several different bacteria. Five bacteria account for nearly all cases in children, however, and each is usually associated with a certain age group. *Escherichia coli* and group B streptococcus cause infection in infants younger than 2 months. *Hemophilus*

Table 9-1 Organisms That Cause Meningitis in Children

Bacteria	*Viruses*
Common	
*Hemophilus influenzae**	Enteroviruses (nonpolio)
Streptococcus pneumoniae	Mumps
Neisseria meningitidis	
Group B streptococcus	
Escherichia coli	
Uncommon	
Listeria monocytogenes	Herpes simplex viruses
Staphylococcus aureus	Arboviruses
Mycobacterium tuberculosis	Lymphocytic choriomeningitis virus
Pseudomonas aeruginosa	Epstein-Barr virus

*Incidence is declining as a result of vaccination of young children.

influenzae type b usually affects children between 6 months and 6 years old. By contrast, *Streptococcus pneumoniae* (pneumococcus) and *Neisseria meningitidis* (meningococcus) are the likely causes of bacterial meningitis in children older than 6 years.

In cases of bacterial meningitis in newborn infants, the infant acquires the bacteria while passing through the birth canal. Older infants or young children typically acquire meningitis-producing bacteria from the mouth or lung secretions of other children or adults. In the susceptible child, the bacteria multiply, usually in the throat, and are then carried by the blood stream to the brain and spinal cord.

Healthy humans are often carriers of bacteria that can cause meningitis. If a susceptible child (ie, one not immune by *H influenzae* vaccination or prior contact with the bacterium) encounters the bacterium, there is a possibility that meningitis or some other form of illness such as middle ear infection (otitis media), infection of joints (septic arthritis), infection around the eye (orbital cellulitis), or infection of the epiglottis (epiglottitis) may occur.

Bacterial meningitis occurs worldwide, but unlike viral meningitis it does not exhibit much seasonal variability. Bacterial meningitis can affect any child, regardless of race or socioeconomic class. Children with certain underlying disorders such as sickle cell anemia, diabetes mellitus, malnutrition, or acquired immunodeficiency syndrome (AIDS) or other abnormalities of the immune system are particularly susceptible.

Signs and Symptoms

The typical signs and symptoms of meningitis are stiff neck (due to inflammation and irritation of the leptomeninges), fever, vomiting, lethargy (inappropriate sleepiness), and a disdain for bright lights (photophobia). Children old enough to talk may also complain of severe headaches.

In the newborn infant, the signs are usually subtle and include irritability, poor feeding, listlessness, pallor, and temperature instability. If the disease progresses rapidly, or if the diagnosis is delayed, the child may have seizures or become comatose. In severe cases of meningitis, shock and death can occur rapidly.

Diagnosis

The diagnosis of meningitis is established by performing a spinal tap (lumbar puncture). This safe and relatively simple procedure involves introducing a thin needle into the spinal canal below the level of the spinal cord and sampling the cerebrospinal fluid (CSF). Normally, CSF appears crystal clear and contains few or no white blood cells. In cases of meningitis, the CSF becomes cloudy and contains numerous white blood cells, a sign of infection or inflammation of the leptomeninges.

Other laboratory tests help determine which virus or bacterium is responsible. In typical cases of bacterial meningitis, the offending bacterium can be grown from samples of CSF (and often blood), usually within 48 hours. In cases of viral meningitis, the agent can sometimes be cultured from CSF, feces, throat washings, or blood. Blood samples drawn during the acute illness and several weeks later during convalescence can be screened for antibodies to specific microorganisms.

Management

The type of treatment given to a child with meningitis depends on whether the disease is caused by a virus, a bacterium, or other agent. Children with viral meningitis typically have a mild, self-limiting illness and do not require antibiotic therapy. More serious cases may require hospitalization and intravenous fluids, but even these infections usually last only a few days and resolve without complications.

Bacterial meningitis, on the other hand, is a life-threatening disease that requires early treatment. The child must be hospitalized and given intravenous antibiotics. Severely ill children may require intensive care therapy.

Prevention by vaccine has become the most effective way of controlling meningitis. The first vaccine for *Hemophilus influenzae* type b, once the most frequent bacterial cause of childhood meningitis, was licensed in 1985. Although this first vaccine was not as beneficial as hoped, subsequent vaccines have effectively protected the vast majority of fully vaccinated children against meningitis due to *H influenzae*. Consequently, the number of cases of *H influenzae* meningitis in the United States has declined dramatically in the 1990s, giving hope that this childhood disease can be eradicated.

Complications

Most cases of viral meningitis are uncomplicated and brief, rarely lasting more than 7 to 10 days. Recovery is usually complete, although some children have residual irritability, muscle pain, and decreased coordination for a few weeks after the acute illness. Some children also complain that they are unable to concentrate on school work. These symptoms are usually transient, and children should be encouraged to return to school as soon as the acute illness subsides.

In contrast to viral meningitis, bacterial meningitis can produce several complications that may have adverse long-term effects on the child. A common early complication is seizures, which occur in approximately 30% of children with bacterial meningitis. Seizures can be generalized throughout the body (grand mal) or involve only an arm or leg on one side of the body (focal). The most serious type is continuous grand mal convulsions (status epilepticus).

Another serious complication of bacterial meningitis is coma. Children who become comatose generally have a less favorable long-term prognosis than children who remain awake. Other early neurologic complications of bacterial meningitis include collections of fluid between the brain and skull (subdural effusions), brain swelling (cerebral edema), stroke, and damage to the eighth cranial nerves, the nerves that control hearing.

Children with bacterial meningitis occasionally develop infections at sites other than the brain or cranial nerves. Relatively common complications include arthritis, pneumonia, and infection of the pericardium, the membrane covering the heart (this condition is known as pericarditis).

Despite appropriate treatment, many children die of bacterial meningitis. Mortality is lowest among children with *Hemophilus influenzae* type b meningitis and highest among newborns with *Escherichia coli* meningitis and older children with pneumococcal meningitis. Death is usually a result of cardiac arrest due to brain swelling or bacteria-induced shock.

Of primary importance to educators are the long-term effects that bacterial meningitis can have on hearing and intelligence. Approximately 10% of the survivors have hearing loss in one or both ears. This hearing loss results from direct damage to the nerve endings in the inner ear. Deafness after bacterial meningitis occurs more often in children who have other serious neurologic deficits, such as mental retardation, seizures, or motor abnormalities. The likelihood of hearing loss can be reduced, however, by treating children early in their illness with the medication dexamethasone. When hearing loss occurs, it is usually permanent.

Bacterial meningitis remains one of the more common causes of acquired (noninherited) mental retardation in children. The children most likely to have intellectual impairments are those who experienced seizures, coma, or shock and those who were younger than 1 year when they contracted the illness. Various degrees of intellectual deficits are found in up to 30% of the survivors of bacterial meningitis. Outcome has generally been least favorable among survivors of neonatal meningitis and most favorable among survivors of childhood *H influenzae* or meningococcal meningitis.

In addition to hearing loss and intellectual deficits, the long-term complications of bacterial meningitis include seizures, motor impairments, and hydrocephalus. Seizures can be of several types, including generalized convulsions (grand mal), staring spells (petit mal), and loss of awareness, often with lip smacking or other unusual repetitive movements (complex partial seizures). Motor impairments consist of increased muscle tone (spasticity) and variable degrees of muscle paralysis. Children occasionally have hydrocephalus, an accumulation of CSF in the brain. This condition may require a shunt or tubing that drains CSF from the brain into the abdomen.

Recommendations

Viral meningitis is typically a benign illness that poses little or no threat to most healthy children or adults. Nonetheless, affected children should be excluded from school or day care environments until acute symptoms (fever and vomiting) subside.

When a case of bacterial meningitis occurs, steps should be taken to prevent the spread of the responsible bacterium. In cases of *H influenzae* or

Neisseria meningitidis meningitis, antibiotic protection (prophylaxis) should be given to children and adults who have had close contact with the affected child (currently, rifampin is the recommended medication for children and nonpregnant adults). Close contacts include household members and children or adults in group day care or nursery schools. Young children between the ages of 6 and 24 months are at greatest risk. Because the organisms are transmitted by oral or respiratory secretions, casual contact—the kind that occurs among school-age children—is generally not considered a sufficient basis for preventive antibiotic. Updated recommendations regarding antibiotic prophylaxis for contacts of meningitis cases are published every 3 to 5 years by the American Academy of Pediatrics. To obtain copies of this material, write the American Academy of Pediatrics, PO Box 927, Elk Grove Village, IL 60007.

When neurologic injury is a result of bacterial meningitis, the child may require early intervention programs, particularly if the handicaps include sensorineural hearing loss (nerve deafness) or developmental delay. Children with hearing loss usually require some type of an aid, and those with severe deafness may need special supportive services throughout the school years. Children with developmental delay or mental retardation require intellectual assessment and appropriate educational placement. Most children who have brain damage from meningitis exhibit mild to moderate delays. Some children have severe retardation, however, with features that resemble autism, including deficient interpersonal skills, impaired language development, and ritualistic behavior.

Seizures can interfere with attention span and memory. Hence the child with poorly controlled seizures poses problems in the classroom. Children with frequent petit mal spells often appear to be daydreaming, although most daydreaming is not seizural. Brief grand mal seizures require only limited first aid, but grand mal seizures that last longer than 5 minutes require medical attention. After a grand mal seizure subsides, children may vomit, complain of headaches or muscle pains, and want to sleep.

Children with motor handicaps or spasticity often require long-term physical therapy. Occasionally, severe spasticity responds to certain muscle-relaxing drugs. Such drugs should be used only under the guidance of a physician who is familiar with their use in children.

ENCEPHALITIS

Encephalitis is an infection or inflammation of brain tissue that is usually caused by a viral agent. Many of the same viruses that cause meningitis can also produce encephalitis. Indeed, children occasionally have features of both illnesses; that is, they have meningoencephalitis. Encephalitis, although relatively infrequent, is a potential cause of long-term neurologic handicaps in children.

Cause

The viral agents most commonly responsible for encephalitis (Table 9-2) are the herpesviruses, the enteroviruses, and the arboviruses (numerous different species of tick- and mosquito-borne viruses that are carried by wild birds, rodents, and other small animals, Table 9-3).

Other viruses that may cause encephalitis are the measles virus, mumps virus, and the adenoviruses. Infections with many potentially encephalitis-producing viruses (such as mumps and measles) have been prevented by vaccination. Rabies virus, although greatly feared, causes few cases of encephalitis in developed countries such as the United States.

Encephalitis is occasionally caused by infectious agents other than viruses. One such agent, known as a rickettsia, is responsible for Rocky Mountain spotted fever, an illness characterized by rash and encephalitis. Two bacterial organisms that can provoke an encephalitic illness are *Leptospira* species and *Mycoplasma pneumoniae*. Meningoencephalitis can also be a complication of Lyme disease (discussed in Chapter 17).

Encephalitis-producing organisms reach the brain in several ways. Most commonly, they first multiply in other tissues, such as the liver or lymph nodes, and then enter the blood stream, which carries the viral particles to the brain. Certain viruses, such as herpes simplex virus, may exist in a hidden (latent) state within the brain tissue and reactivate spontaneously to produce symptoms of encephalitis.

The rabies virus invades the skin from the saliva of the infected animal and enters human nerves, which transmit the virus to the spinal cord and

Table 9-2 Organisms That Cause Encephalitis in Children

Viruses	*Nonviral organisms*
Herpes simplex virus	Rickettsia species (Rocky Mountain spotted fever)
Arboviruses (many)	Spirochetes (Lyme disease and syphilis)
Measles virus	Parasites (*Toxoplasma gondii,* amebae, malaria)
Mumps virus	Other (*Mycoplasma pneumoniae*)
Epstein-Barr virus	
Enteroviruses	
Adenoviruses	
Rabies virus	

Table 9-3 Epidemiology of Meningoencephalitis in North America

Disease	*Vector*	*Season*	*Location*	*Age*
Herpes encephalitis	None*	Any	Widespread	Any
California encephalitis	Mosquito	Summer	Midwest US	5–15 years
Lyme disease	Tick	Summer	Northern US	Any
Rocky Mountain spotted fever	Tick	Summer	South-central, eastern US	Any
Mycoplasma pneumoniae	None*	Any	Widespread	Any
Chickenpox	None*	Winter, spring	Widespread	Children
Western equine encephalitis	Mosquito	Summer	Western US	Any
St Louis encephalitis	Mosquito	Summer	Central US	Any
Eastern equine encephalitis	Mosquito	Summer	Eastern, Gulf coast US	Any
Rabies†	Mammals‡	Any	Widespread	Any

*Spread by human-to-human contact.
†Fewer than five cases per year in the United States.
‡Many animals can be infected; raccoons, skunks, and bats are important reservoirs of the rabies virus.

brain. As a result of this unique mode of travel, the incubation period for rabies is usually 1 to 2 months and sometimes even longer. Tick- or mosquito-borne arboviruses are inoculated into the skin or muscle, where they multiply before entering the blood stream; these have a much shorter incubation period.

Encephalitis occurs in children throughout the world. As their names imply, certain types of encephalitis (eg, Japanese encephalitis) cluster in geographic (endemic) regions. Names can be deceiving, however. California encephalitis, although originally detected in the state of California, is most common in the midwest. Most cases of Rocky Mountain spotted fever are reported in the southeastern or south-central states rather than in the Rocky Mountain states. These geographic variations result from the unique distributions of mosquitos or ticks (vectors of transmission) and animal reservoirs.

Encephalitis-causing viruses generally exhibit seasonal variability. For example, mumps virus infections are more common in late winter or early spring, and the enteroviral illnesses are more likely to occur in summer or fall. Tick- and mosquito-borne encephalitis occurs in warm months, when these insects are active (epidemics may result from conditions that favor breeding of mosquitos, such as excessive rainfall and irrigation). An im-

Color Plates

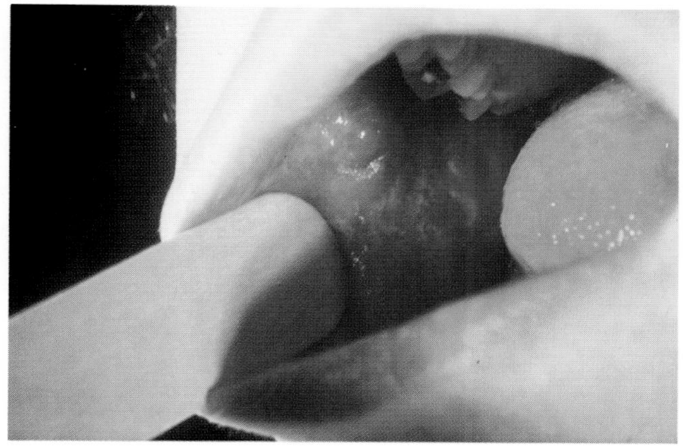

Plate 1 Thrush (oral candidiasis)

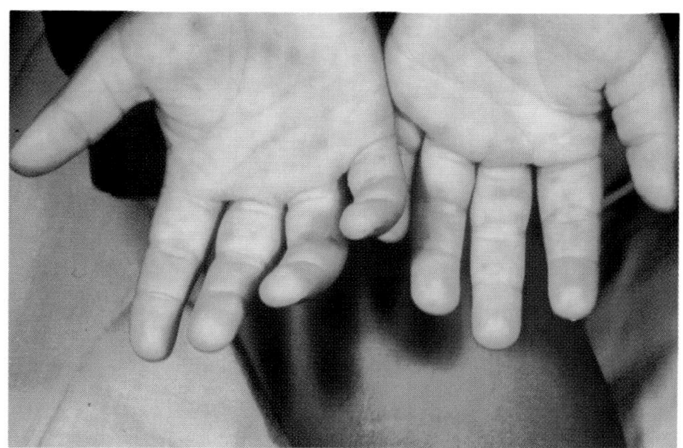

Plate 2a Hand, foot, and mouth disease

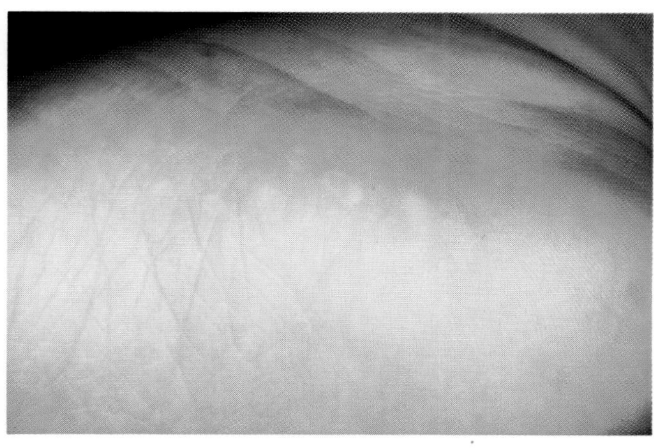

Plate 2b Hand, foot, and mouth disease

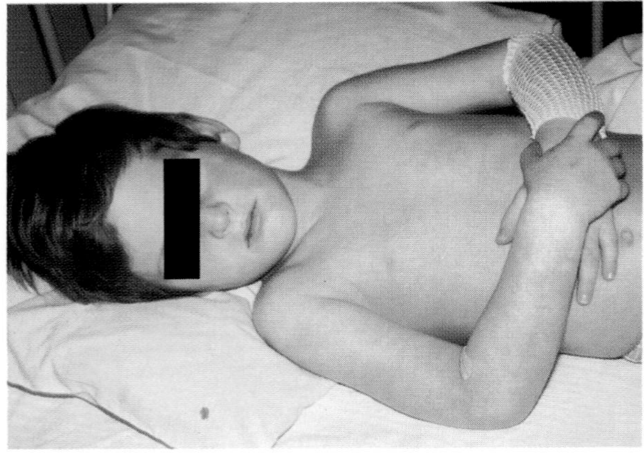

Plate 3 Scarlet fever

Plate 4a Chicken pox (varicella)

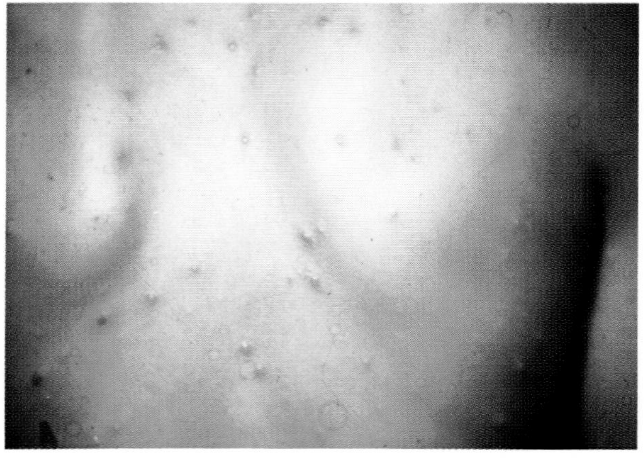

Plate 4b Chicken pox (varicella)

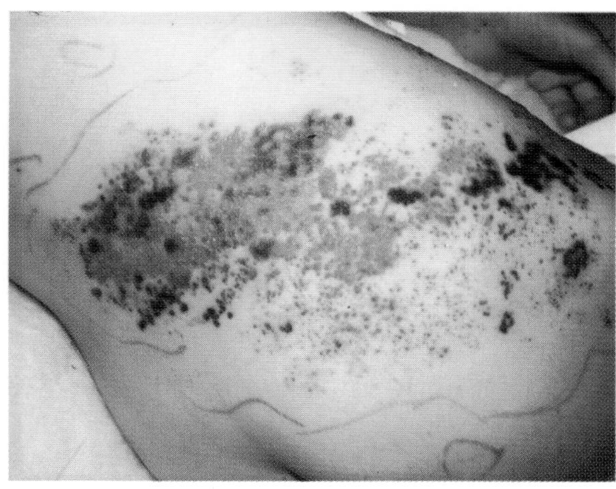

Plate 5 Shingles (zoster)

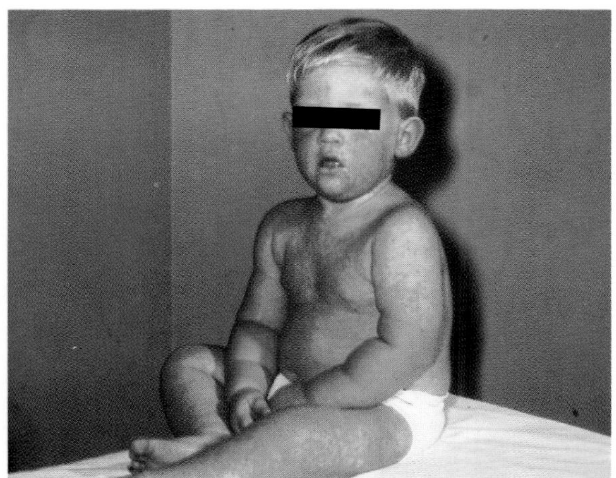

Plate 6a Measles

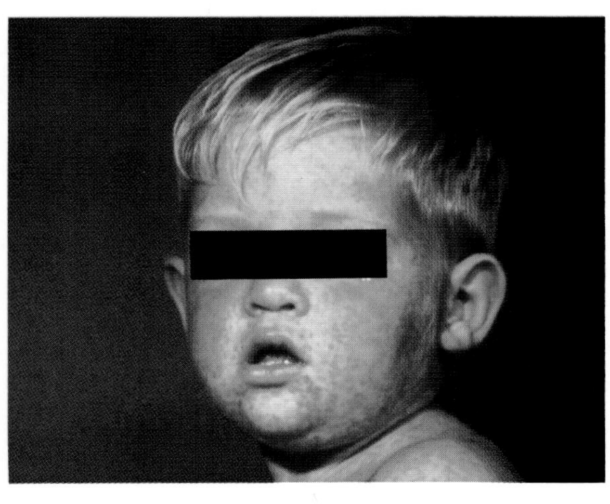

Plate 6b Measles

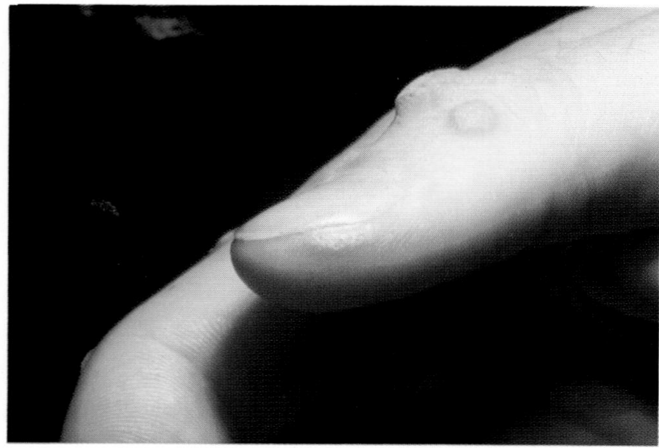

Plate 7 Warts

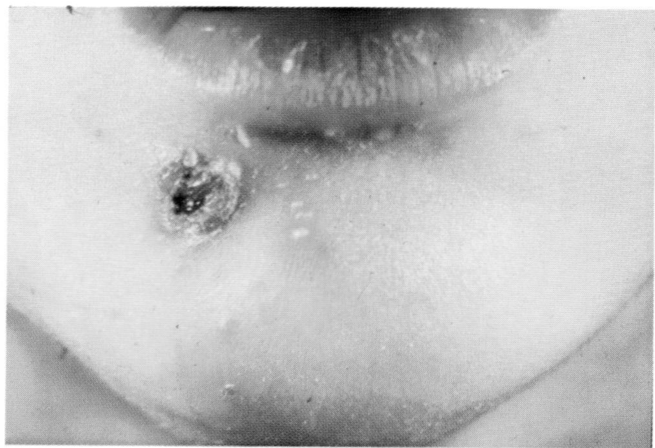

Plate 8 Impetigo

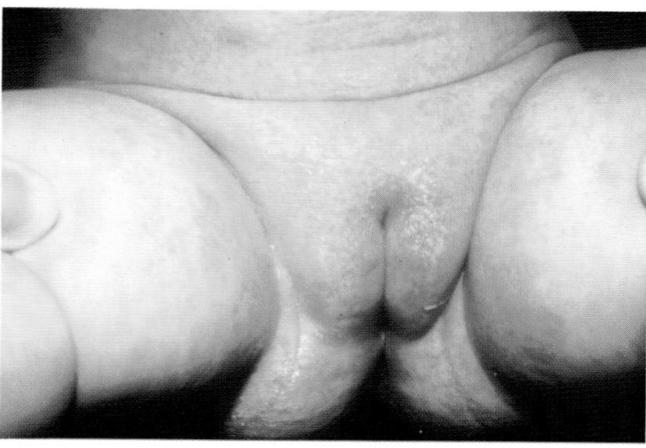

Plate 9 Diaper rash due to candidiasis

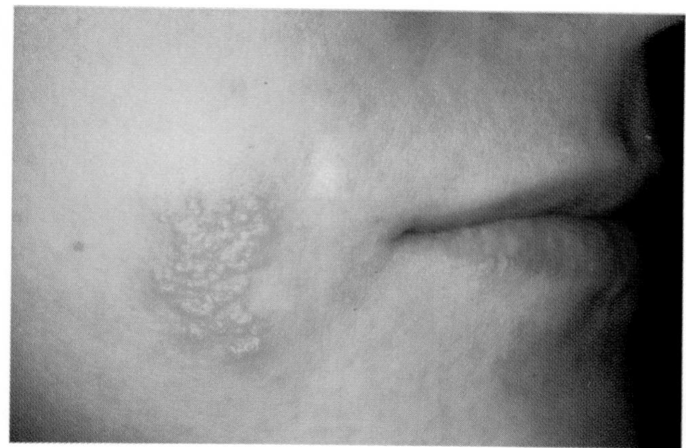

Plate 10 Herpes Simplex Virus Infection

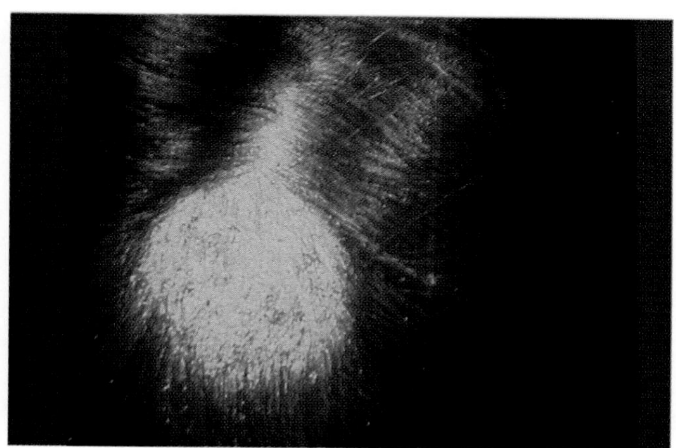

Plate 11 Ringworm of the Scalp (*tinea capitis*)

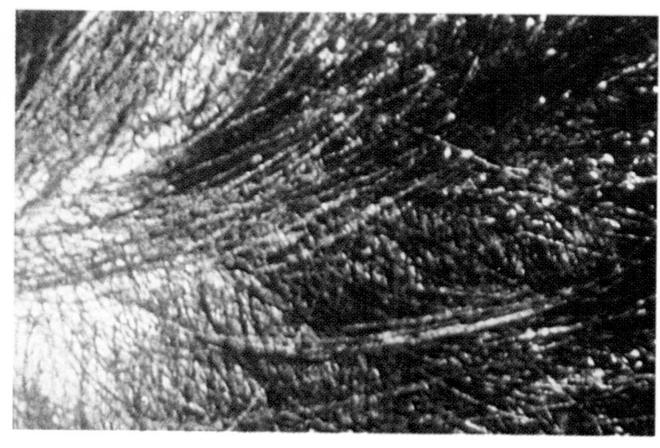

Plate 12 Nits

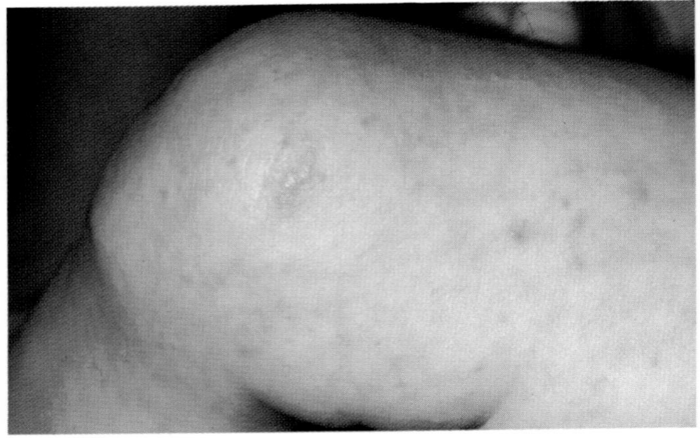

Plate 13 Scabies

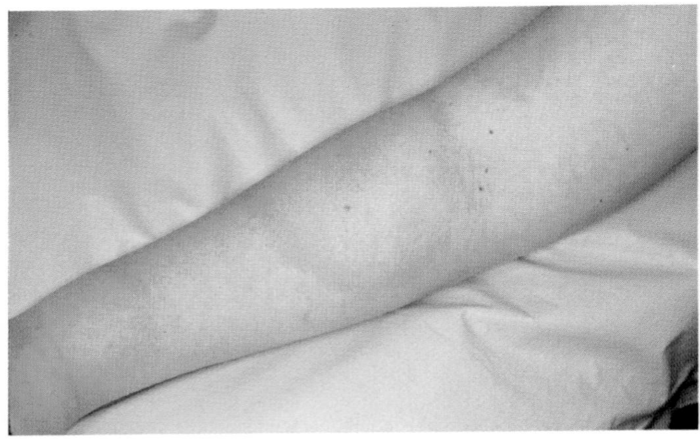

Plate 14 Rash associated with Lyme disease

Source: Courtesy of Dr. Mary Jones, The University of Iowa College of Medicine.

portant virus that displays no seasonal variation is herpes simplex virus type 1, the most common cause of the nonepidemic form of encephalitis.

Exactly why encephalitis develops in one person and not another is not completely understood. Most affected persons are otherwise healthy and do not have obvious factors that predispose to encephalitis. Although most persons with encephalitis do not have underlying medical conditions, persons with disorders such as AIDS, which impairs the body's immune mechanisms, clearly are at increased risk of acquiring certain types of encephalitis. Age appears to be an important factor because attack rates (rate of disease per susceptible individual) are highest in infants and the elderly. Occupational or recreational factors also contribute because the arthropod-borne diseases require exposure to the infected tick or mosquito.

Signs and Symptoms

The signs and symptoms of encephalitis suggest involvement of brain tissue. They include reduced alertness, seizures, or localized neurologic abnormalities (eg, paralysis of an arm or leg), all of which occur relatively early in the course of the illness. Seizures may be repetitive, and coma can develop rapidly. Swelling of brain tissue frequently leads to further injury of vital areas of the brain.

Children usually have high fever and may have other systemic signs. Children with encephalitis due to measles, chickenpox, Lyme disease, or Rocky Mountain spotted fever, as examples, typically exhibit skin rashes. Enlargement of the salivary glands typically precedes or accompanies mumps meningoencephalitis, and enlargement of the spleen or liver can occur during Epstein-Barr virus infection (infectious mononucleosis).

Diagnosis

Diagnostic techniques to help confirm encephalitis include a brain wave test [electroencephalogram (EEG)], a brain imaging study [either a magnetic resonance imaging (MRI) or a computed tomographic (CT) scan], and a spinal tap. In a child with encephalitis, the EEG usually reveals slowing of brain wave activity or seizure discharges. The CT scan may be normal or show localized brain abnormalities (characteristic of herpes simplex virus encephalitis) or brain swelling. The CSF usually shows signs of infection, including increased numbers of white blood cells.

Identifying the viral cause of encephalitis is often difficult. In the first place, viruses may not be present in the CSF (few patients with herpes simplex virus type 1 encephalitis have this virus in their CSF, for example). Feces, throat secretions, or blood can yield viruses in some patients, however, especially those with enteroviral diseases. In certain instances, particularly in suspected cases of herpes encephalitis, a biopsy of brain tissue (a delicate but usually safe procedure) is the only effective method of obtaining the virus.

Another problem in identifying the specific organism is that culturing viruses requires a highly specialized laboratory, available only at a tertiary medical center or a reference laboratory. Blood tests for antibodies to viral agents are useful in selected cases of encephalitis, but these are time consuming and usually not beneficial during the early phase of an encephalitic illness. Even when the testing is thorough, no cause is identified in 25% to 50% of encephalitis cases.

In certain cases, a careful history of travel or exposures can help pinpoint the diagnosis. For example, a tick bite in a child who develops signs of meningoencephalitis suggests Lyme disease or Rocky Mountain spotted fever. Similarly, a recent animal bite raises the question of rabies.

Management

In most cases of viral encephalitis, treatment consists solely of supportive care. Repetitive or prolonged seizures may require therapy with an anticonvulsant medication. The comatose child requires intravenous fluids and close attention to important body functions, such as breathing, urine production, and heart activity.

Specific antiviral medication is currently available only for a few disorders. Persons who have encephalitis due to herpes simplex virus or varicella zoster virus (the chickenpox virus) often improve during treatment with the antiviral drug acyclovir, which acts selectively on infected cells. Despite antiviral drug therapy, however, mortality due to herpes encephalitis still averages approximately 25%.

Encephalitis caused by organisms other than viruses can occasionally be treated with conventional antibiotic medications. For example, children with Rocky Mountain spotted fever typically improve dramatically during therapy with chloramphenicol or tetracycline, and mycoplasma infections usually respond to erythromycin or tetracycline. In contrast, there is no effective drug for rabies virus and equine virus encephalitis.

Vaccines have been developed for certain types of encephalitis, such as Japanese encephalitis, and their use has substantially reduced the numbers of encephalitis cases in endemic areas of the world. Vaccination against the rabies virus has virtually eliminated rabies among domestic dogs and cats in the United States, and the current human vaccines and immune globulin are highly effective in preventing disease in humans bitten by rabid animals.

Complications

The complications of encephalitis vary greatly and depend on such factors as the age of the child, the severity of the illness, and the causative agent. Young infants tend to be more susceptible to encephalitis and often have more severe encephalitic illness than older children. As a result, the incidence of death or long-term complications is greater for this age group.

Encephalitis that is caused by mumps virus or the enteroviruses is generally mild and without complications. Rarely does it result in death. Occasionally, a child who recovers from mumps meningoencephalitis develops hearing loss or hydrocephalus due to inflammation of CSF pathways.

The prognosis for children who acquire mosquito-borne viral encephalitis is quite variable. California encephalitis has a low mortality rate, although some children who recover from this form of encephalitis have learning or emotional difficulties. Western equine encephalitis carries a mortality rate of approximately 10%, and a substantial proportion of childhood survivors have neurologic handicaps, including seizures, behavioral changes, mental retardation, and motor deficits. Mortality rates for Eastern equine encephalitis, a rare disorder, approach 50%, and most survivors have residual neurologic deficits.

Age and severity of illness play an important role in determining the outcome of children with herpes simplex virus encephalitis. Neonates who survive herpes simplex virus infections (usually due to herpes simplex virus type 2) often have serious, long-term handicaps. Older children with herpes simplex virus type 1 encephalitis generally fare better, although many survivors have important neurobehavioral deficits, including seizures, motor deficits, personality disorders, memory loss, and variable degrees of cognitive dysfunction.

Some survivors of chickenpox encephalitis have neurologic handicaps, such as seizures, mental retardation, or motor deficits. Chickenpox-related infection or inflammation of the cerebellum, the portion of the brain responsible for fine control of body movements, may also cause a disturbance of balance and coordination (ataxia).

Recommendations

Although many serious cases, such as herpes simplex virus type 1 encephalitis or tick- or mosquito-borne encephalitis, are not spread by person-to-person contact, encephalitis should be regarded as a potentially communicable disease. Affected children should be isolated from others until the cause of the illness can be determined. No medications are available to prevent encephalitis.

Some mosquito-borne encephalitides can be prevented by mosquito abatement measures, including the use of insecticides and elimination of breeding areas. These measures may not be completely effective, however, particularly when many different species of mosquitos transmit the offending virus. Often, the most effective way to prevent mosquito-borne encephalitis during rare outbreaks of arboviral illnesses is to protect the child against all mosquito bites. The child should be clothed to reduce the amount of exposed skin, and insect repellants should be applied liberally. Open windows should have screens in place. In addition, outdoor activities should be curtailed in the early morning or evening hours, when mosquitos are active.

Although cases of rabies encephalitis in humans are now rare in most developed nations, rabies remains prevalent in many animal species, both wild and domesticated. When an animal bite occurs, the wound should be cleansed with soap and rinsed generously with water or an antiseptic, and the child should be examined by a physician to determine whether suturing is necessary. The animal should be captured and observed for illness (if a cat or dog) or killed for rabies studies of the brain. Skunks (wild), foxes, raccoons, and bats should always be regarded as rabid. If rabies prophylaxis is deemed necessary, the child will receive a combination of antirabies serum and rabies vaccine. The currently available vaccine, produced in human cells, does not have the potentially severe side effects of earlier vaccines. Updated recommendations regarding possible rabies exposure or prophylaxis can be obtained from local or state health departments.

Survivors of encephalitis often require specialized educational services. Early intervention programs may be necessary for young children with developmental delays. Formal cognitive evaluation by a psychologist is beneficial, particularly when school performance does not meet expectations.

BRAIN ABSCESS

Brain abscess is a serious and potentially fatal infection of a localized area of brain tissue. This condition is much less common than either meningitis or encephalitis.

Cause

Brain abscesses can be caused by bacteria, fungi, or parasites. More than 20 different species of bacteria have been associated with brain abscesses in children, and brain abscesses in a single patient frequently contain more than one species of bacteria.

Most children who develop brain abscesses have underlying conditions that predispose them to this infection. One of the most common is congenital heart disease, which may allow the blood to bypass the normal filtering mechanisms of the lung, enabling bacteria or other abscess-producing organisms to reach brain tissue. Children with certain types of heart disease may also have microscopic areas of brain injury (stroke) that can become a focus for abscess formation. Children with AIDS have an increased risk of brain abscess, especially abscesses due to parasites such as *Toxoplasma gondii*. Other conditions that can predispose children to brain abscess include chronic infections of the ears or sinuses (sinusitis).

Signs and Symptoms

Most children with brain abscess have headache and alterations of personality or consciousness. Also typical are vomiting, seizures, and localized neurologic signs, such as the inability to use an arm or leg or to see objects in certain fields of vision. Fever is not always present. Young infants may exhibit rapid enlargement of the head and bulging of the soft spot (fontanelle). Some children, particularly those with underlying disorders, may deteriorate rapidly. Death may result from massive swelling of the brain tissue adjacent to the abscess.

Diagnosis

The most effective way to determine whether a child has a brain abscess is to perform an MRI or a CT scan. The vast majority of brain abscesses large enough to produce symptoms can be identified with these techniques.

Even though CSF is abnormal in most children with brain abscess, a spinal tap is not usually performed in these children because it can disrupt pressure relationships within the brain, causing compression of vital areas (a condition referred to as brain herniation).

Management

Most large brain abscesses require drainage by a skilled neurosurgeon. In addition, antibiotics are given intravenously. Response to treatment is generally assessed by frequent neurologic examinations and by repeating the CT scan at intervals.

Complications

Many children have acute complications, including seizures and brain swelling. Seizures are treated with anticonvulsants, such as phenytoin (Dilantin) or phenobarbital. Serious brain swelling must be reduced with such methods as rapid machine-assisted breathing (hyperventilation) or certain medications.

Despite surgery, antibiotics, and measures to reduce brain swelling, between 10% and 30% of children with brain abscesses die. Some studies suggest that at least 70% of the children who survive brain abscess have seizures and that at least 50% have problems with school performance. Another long-term complication of this infection is motor abnormalities, such as alterations in muscle tone and limb paralysis.

Recommendations

Brain abscess is not a communicable disease, and therefore precautionary measures need not be instituted for contacts of affected children. Children who recover from brain abscesses commonly have intellectual deficits, motor abnormalities, and other neurologic problems, all of which require special diagnostic and educational interventions.

REFERENCES

Bale JF Jr. Viral encephalitis. *Med Clin North Am*. 1993; 77:25–42.

Johnson RT. *Viral Infections of the Nervous System*. New York, NY: Raven; 1982.

Kaplan SL. Current management of common bacterial meningitides. *Pediatr Rev*. 1985; 7:77–87.

Chapter 10

Respiratory Illnesses

Respiratory infections include a wide spectrum of problems, ranging from the common cold to life-threatening illnesses. Together they represent the most common diseases of children. Although these infections are often not limited to a single area of the respiratory tract, it is convenient to categorize them according to the area affected most: the nose and throat, the airways, or the lungs.

NOSE AND THROAT (UPPER RESPIRATORY) INFECTIONS

The most prevalent infection of the nose and throat is, of course, the common cold. Although a sore throat often accompanies a cold, it is also a primary symptom of other, potentially more important illness, such as strep throat and infectious mononucleosis.

The Common Cold

The term *common cold* generally refers to upper respiratory (nose and throat) infection caused by viruses and characterized by runny nose (rhinorrhea), nasal congestion, sore throat (pharyngitis), and variable degrees of malaise, fever, or cough.

Cause

Most colds, with or without sore throats, are caused by viruses. The two agents most commonly responsible are rhinoviruses and coronaviruses, which generally produce symptoms limited to the upper respiratory tract.

Other viruses, such as parainfluenza viruses and adenoviruses, can also produce symptoms in the nose and throat, but they more commonly involve the airways or lungs.

Signs and Symptoms

The familiar symptoms of the common cold include runny nose (rhinorrhea), sore throat, malaise, fever (more common in children than in adults), cough, nasal congestion, and headache.

Coldlike symptoms may signal problems other than the common cold and sore throat. A runny nose, for example, can be a manifestation of an allergy. A sore throat is a much less common type of allergic reaction. A sore throat can also be an early sign of *Mycoplasma pneumoniae* infection (although the diagnosis is not made until later, when other symptoms occur). A severe sore throat is also a symptom of diphtheria, a disease that, because of immunization, is exceedingly rare in the United States.

Diagnosis

There are two central issues in diagnosing the common cold. The first is whether the child has a sore (or obviously red) throat. If so, the possibility of strep throat must be excluded by throat culture because this disorder cannot be distinguished from a viral sore throat solely on the basis of appearance. The second important issue is whether the symptoms primarily involve the nose and throat. If coughing is prominent, for example, other lower respiratory illness may be present.

Distinguishing between upper and lower respiratory infections is difficult in children younger than 1 year. Moreover, the same common cold virus that causes no more than a runny nose in an adult can cause high fever and irritability in an infant. Most children who have a common cold without sore throat and who appear well, however, need no diagnostic tests or medical attention, except perhaps for guidance about symptom relief.

Management

Cold remedies are directed at alleviating the symptoms; they do not affect the natural course of the infection. It is appropriate to use whatever medications are helpful for discomfort and fever, provided that the side effects are not worse than the symptoms. Approaches to treatment may change as new symptoms or signs emerge. For example, although the common cold is caused by a virus and does not respond to antibiotics, it may be followed by a middle ear infection (see Chapter 8) or pneumonia, both of which usually require antibiotic treatment.

Complications

Colds are sometimes followed by secondary bacterial infections, probably because of congestion in the adjacent structures: the middle ear, sinuses, and lungs. In the young infant, middle ear infection is the most common complication (see Chapter 8). Sinusitis can also follow colds, although the relatively undeveloped sinuses of young children help reduce this problem. Finally, colds can sometimes lead to pneumonia in children. This complication, however, is more common among the elderly.

Recommendations

Viruses that cause colds are present in the nasal and oral secretions and are transmitted by coughing, sneezing, or direct contact. Beyond infancy, most children with the common cold do not receive medical treatment and continue to attend school or day care. These children are likely to be contagious for several days, not only while fever is present but also early in convalescence. It is impractical, however, to wait until all signs and symptoms have disappeared before allowing reentry. Many children feel well enough to attend school or day care long before the runny nose and cough are gone. Moreover, the usually benign consequences to other children, the ubiquitous character of these viruses, and their virtually routine transmission among children make restrictive policies burdensome. One convenient but crude marker of a higher level of contagion is the presence of fever. Once fever has disappeared, reentry is usually recommended.

Cold-causing viruses are often present on the hands. Proper hand washing is a good way to prevent spread of these viruses.

Although it is not generally desirable or feasible to restrict interactions among children with the common cold, ideally infants younger than 6 months should not have repeated contacts with numerous affected children. This is not because these infants are particularly vulnerable to most respiratory infections but because several of the agents responsible for coldlike illness (such as respiratory syncytial virus and *Bordetella pertussis*) can cause serious lower respiratory tract illness in the early months of life. Also, fever in the early weeks of life, even when related to an apparent cold, mandates more extensive and invasive diagnostic testing.

Strep Throat

Strep throat is a sore or obviously red throat caused by the bacterium group A streptococcus. Strep throat itself is sometimes no more severe than the viral sore throat that accompanies the common cold, but it can be followed by two more serious strep-related illnesses: rheumatic fever and poststreptococcal glomerulonephritis, a kidney disease.

Cause

Strep throat is caused by the bacterium group A streptococcus (*Streptococcus pyogenes*), the same organism responsible for streptococcal lymph vessel infection (sometimes called blood poisoning), impetigo (see Chapter 13), and occasional cases of pneumonia.

Diagnosis

Children who have a sore throat should be tested for group A streptococcal infection. The most common diagnostic technique is the throat culture, which takes 24 hours to complete, although other tests are available that can provide diagnosis in a matter of minutes. These rapid tests have proved reliable enough for presumptive diagnosis and treatment.

Signs and Symptoms

Symptoms of strep throat include sore throat and variable degrees of tonsil swelling, nasal congestion, and fever. Occasionally, a bright red rash is also present, in which case the illness is known as scarlet fever (see Color Plate 3).

Management

Children with proven strep throat are treated with penicillin (or an alternative antibiotic if they are allergic to penicillin). Although antibiotic therapy may hasten resolution of the sore throat, the primary therapeutic goal is preventing rheumatic fever. Penicillin therapy can be given orally or by injection. If oral, it should be continued for a full 10 days, even if symptoms disappear sooner. The full course of therapy is the best way to prevent rheumatic fever. In most but not all instances, the streptococcal bacteria are eradicated from the throat by antibiotic treatment.

Complications

Two conditions that can follow strep throat are rheumatic fever and poststreptococcal glomerulonephritis. Rheumatic fever, an inflammatory condition of the heart and other tissues (especially the joints), is not a direct streptococcal infection of the heart but an immune reaction within the heart. Penicillin therapy of strep throat has helped make this condition uncommon in the United States. Children who have recovered from rheumatic fever receive continuous penicillin to prevent recurrence (see Chapter 17).

Poststreptococcal glomerulonephritis is an uncommon inflammatory condition that affects primarily the kidneys. Like rheumatic fever, it results from an immune reaction. Most children with this complication recover fully.

Another, less serious strep-related condition is scarlet fever, a term used less commonly today than in the past. The ominous-sounding name usually implies little more than strep throat accompanied by a rash of sandpaper texture that is most prominent over the upper chest, head, and neck.

Finally, since the late 1980s, severe, sometimes fatal streptococcal disease has been observed more frequently. Although uncommon, these cases have caused concern among health care professionals because of the rapidity of progression, the invasive and serious character of the infection, and the slow response to penicillin.

Recommendations

Children treated for strep throat are generally presumed to be noncontagious 24 hours after penicillin therapy is begun.

Infectious Mononucleosis

Infectious mononucleosis, often called mono, is a usually mild viral infection that results in a complex of signs and symptoms including sore throat, fatigue, swollen lymph glands, fever, and an enlarged liver and spleen.

Cause

This condition is caused by the Epstein-Barr virus, one of the herpesviruses of human importance. It is found in and transmitted by respiratory secretions.

Signs and Symptoms

Infectious mononucleosis is often characterized by sore throat, malaise, and fever. These symptoms are frequently compounded by swollen tonsils, swollen lymph nodes in the neck area, and an enlarged liver and spleen. There may also be inflammation of the liver (hepatitis). Fatigue is highly variable and less likely to be prolonged in the young child than in the adolescent or adult. Indeed, all these symptoms tend to be mild or absent in young children, a fact that once led physicians to believe that this infection was relatively rare in this age group.

Diagnosis

Infectious mononucleosis is usually detected by two tests. One is a microscopic examination of the blood smear. In the child with mononucleosis, this usually reveals changes in the shape and texture of certain white blood cells. The second test, a screening for certain blood proteins (heterophile), is reliable for older children but likely to be falsely negative during the preschool years.

Management

In the early stages of mononucleosis, the primary management strategy is rest. Many physicians feel that physical exertion and stress may prolong the course of symptoms or precipitate relapse. This appears to be more of a problem in adolescents or young adults, many of whom complain of fatigue with or without exertion weeks or months after the onset of symptoms.

Complications

Complications of infectious mononucleosis are uncommon They include meningoencephalitis (see Chapter 9), which usually resolves quickly and spontaneously; a narrowed air passage, caused by tonsil enlargement (which can be decreased rapidly with steroid drugs); and a ruptured spleen, which is preventable by avoiding trauma to the enlarged spleen.

Recommendations

Children with infectious mononucleosis can reenter day care or school as soon as symptoms subside and they are feeling well. Most young children do not require restriction of activities. Children with enlarged spleens, however, should not participate in contact sports.

AIRWAYS INFECTIONS

The airways are common targets for many infectious agents, including those responsible for croup, epiglottitis, bronchiolitis, and whooping cough (Table 10-1).

Croup

Croup is a term frequently applied to the common viral infections of the larynx (voice box), trachea (windpipe), and bronchi (large airways). More precise terms for croup are laryngitis (involving the larynx), laryngotracheitis (involving the larynx and trachea), and laryngotracheobronchitis (involving the larynx, trachea, and bronchi). Because the larynx contains the vocal cords, croup is characterized by a hoarse, barking cough.

Table 10-1 Causative Agents in Common Airways Infections

Infection	*Causative agent*
Croup	Parainfluenza virus (most common) Influenza virus Adenovirus Respiratory syncytial virus
Epiglottitis	*Hemophilus influenzae* type b*
Bronchiolitis	Respiratory syncytial virus Parainfluenza virus Other respiratory viruses
Whooping cough (pertussis)	*Bordetella pertussis**

*Bacterial and therefore treatable with certain antibiotics.

Cause

Croup is caused by a number of respiratory viruses, including parainfluenza virus (the major cause), influenza virus, adenovirus, and respiratory syncytial virus.

Signs and Symptoms

Croup is characterized by a barking cough and stridor, the coarse breathing noise that is produced by a narrowing of the large air passages. Stridor that is accompanied by an apparent air hunger may signal epiglottitis, a far more serious condition in which swelling around the epiglottis can rapidly block off air completely.

Diagnosis

A diagnosis of croup is based on history and physical examination. The most critical diagnostic problem is distinguishing probable croup from the life-threatening condition epiglottitis. Croup usually waxes and wanes over a period of several days, whereas epiglottitis generally progresses rapidly. Other family members are more likely to have had recent respiratory infections with croup than with epiglottitis. Also, a child with croup appears less ill or anxious than a child with epiglottitis.

Blood tests and cultures cannot provide a definitive diagnosis of croup, although the white blood cell profile may indicate a viral agent, thereby helping distinguish croup from the bacterial infection epiglottitis.

Management

Croup is usually managed by treating the symptoms, particularly by moisturizing the air. Some children have sufficiently labored breathing to warrant hospitalization and mist tents; a few require more vigorous respiratory support and placement of an endotracheal tube in the major airway. Hospital therapy for croup may also include inhaled medications to reduce airways symptoms.

Complications

Croup is sometimes complicated by bacterial pneumonia.

Recommendations

Croup is about as contagious as the common cold. At least several days of contagion should be presumed, but children need not be excluded from school or day care simply because of a lingering cough. Ideally, children with croup or other respiratory infections should not have close contact with infants younger than 6 months.

Epiglottitis

Epiglottitis is a bacterial infection characterized by a life-threatening swelling of the epiglottis, the structure that acts as a kind of swinging door to the trachea. This relatively uncommon disease affects children of all ages and requires emergency treatment and hospitalization.

Cause

Epiglottitis is usually caused by the bacterium *Hemophilus influenzae* type b.

Signs and Symptoms

Increased swelling around the epiglottis blocks the upper airways, producing gasping or otherwise apparent air hunger. The child appears flushed, ill, and apprehensive, often breathing and moving carefully. Typically, the illness develops rapidly. Without emergency medical treatment, the airway may close completely within hours.

Diagnosis

Physicians suspecting epiglottitis do not examine the epiglottis until a specialized medical team is assembled that can manage the airway in a controlled setting, such as an operating room. A red and swollen epiglottis provides the presumptive diagnosis. The usual cause of epiglottis is the bacterium *H influenzae* type b, which can be cultured from the area. Some physicians also obtain radiographs of the neck.

Management

Epiglottitis requires the immediate assembly of a team capable of establishing an artificial airway. In most cases, a tube is inserted into the airway through the nose or mouth; if the swelling is too great, however, the tube may be inserted into the windpipe through a skin incision (this procedure is called a tracheostomy). After an airway is established, the child is given antibiotics and, possibly, antiinflammatory agents.

Complications

The most serious complication of epiglottitis is complete obstruction of air flow by the swollen epiglottis. Unless an airway can be established quickly, this complication can lead to death.

Recommendations

Whenever a serious disease occurs, parents and caretakers understandably become alarmed about contagion. With epiglottitis, however, there is limited risk of spread. It is important to note that the causative organism may produce other diseases, such as meningitis, at a low rate in susceptible contacts. Equally important is the fact that the *H influenzae* type b vaccine is effectively reducing *Hemophilus*-related diseases and is likely to make epiglottitis even more rare than in the past. Household and day care contacts of children with epiglottitis should be treated the same as persons exposed to other types of disease caused by *H influenzae* type b (see Chapter 5).

Bronchiolitis

Bronchiolitis is an inflammation of the bronchioles, structures that convey air between the major airways (bronchi) and tiny air sacs (alveoli). This viral infection generally affects young infants, who often require hospitalization.

Cause

More than half of all cases of bronchiolitis are caused by the respiratory syncytial virus. The parainfluenza virus is another agent that can cause this disease.

Signs and Symptoms

Bronchiolitis generally produces signs and symptoms relating to the lower airways, including wheezing, increased rate of respiration, and small airways crackles caused by congestion of the bronchioles (audible with a stethoscope).

Diagnosis

Diagnosis is based on history and physical examination. Rapid diagnostic tests and culture for respiratory syncytial virus and other viruses can help substantiate the diagnosis, but these are not widely available.

Management

Treatment consists largely of supportive measures, such as oxygen, rather than antibiotics or antiviral drugs. The drug ribavirin has proven helpful for children who have serious bronchiolitis due to respiratory syncytial virus, particularly those with underlying heart and lung conditions.

Complications

Bronchiolitis is sometimes followed by bacterial pneumonia, possibly because of bronchiole congestion.

Recommendations

Bronchiolitis, especially if caused by respiratory syncytial virus, is generally contagious for 1 or 2 weeks. During this time, contacts with other children, particularly infants younger than 6 months, should be restricted.

Whooping Cough

Whooping cough (pertussis) is a serious and sometimes fatal infection of the large airways. It is often characterized by a whoop, which occurs when the child rapidly inhales after a series of coughing exhalations. The incidence of this disease, which affects primarily young children, declined dramatically after the 1930s, largely as a result of mass immunization. Nonetheless, whooping cough continues to occur every year in nearly every state in the United States, often resulting in prolonged hospitalization or death, particularly in young infants.

Cause

Whooping cough is caused by the bacterium *Bordetella pertussis.*

Signs and Symptoms

Whooping cough is most notable for the duration of its symptoms, which often last 6 to 8 weeks. The first weeks (catarrhal phase) are usually characterized by runny nose, low-grade fever, and other upper respiratory symptoms. The second (paroxysmal) phase may last several weeks and is characterized by severe coughing episodes. The third and final (convalescent) phase may also last several weeks, during which time the coughing episodes become progressively milder and less frequent.

Diagnosis

Diagnosis is initially based on history and physical examination. The protracted course of this disease and the classic whoop arouse suspicion, which may be supported by the complete blood count (whooping cough produces high elevations of blood lymphocytes). Rapid diagnostic tests for the bacterium *Bordetella pertussis* in respiratory secretions often provide a presumptive diagnosis within 24 hours. These tests are not widely available, however. Cultures can provide definitive proof of the agent, but they require special techniques that also are not widely available.

Management

Whooping cough often requires hospitalization, especially in infants, because coughing episodes are often severe and may persist for weeks or even months. The antibiotic erythromycin is generally given for 14 days, both to the patient and to household contacts, to eradicate the responsible organism.

Complications

The most common complication of whooping cough is pneumonia. The coughing episodes can also cause bursting of tiny blood vessels in the skin, particularly in the face.

Despite modern intensive care, a small percentage of infants continue to die of the respiratory complications of whooping cough, a fact that must not be forgotten when one is formulating immunization policies. The risk of death or prolonged hospitalization with this disease far outweighs that of vaccine side effects (see Chapter 3).

Recommendations

When a child is diagnosed as having whooping cough, efforts should be made to identify possible sources and to prevent contagion in contacts. Parents of young children who have come into contact with this disease should consult their physician or public health authorities regarding vaccine boosters (in immunized children) and antibiotics (usually erythromycin) to prevent illness. The greatest risk for serious disease is in the young infant. Educators and child care providers who encounter unimmunized children should be aware of the dangers of pertussis.

PNEUMONIA AND OTHER LUNG INFECTIONS

Pneumonia

Pneumonia is an infection of the lung tissue caused by many types of microorganisms, including viruses, bacteria, and chlamydia and mycoplasma species. The term *pneumonia* is sometimes used interchangeably with *pneumonitis*, which actually means inflammation (infectious or otherwise) of the lung. Pneumonia often occurs during or after upper respiratory or airways infections. Factors that may influence the likelihood of this disease include age, general health, and immune status. A chronically ill child with an upper respiratory infection is much more likely to develop pneumonia than a healthy school-age child. Children experience pneumonia frequently enough, however, to warrant a detailed discussion of this disease.

Cause

Because lung infections are located deep within the body, they are not easily accessible for culture. Thus the causative organism is often unidentified when treatment is begun, and the pneumonia is categorized as presumed viral, presumed bacterial, presumed mycoplasmal, and so forth.

Some viruses, including cytomegalovirus (see Chapter 14), seldom cause pneumonia unless there are unusual circumstances, such as when normal immune defense is impaired. The adenovirus, on the other hand, occasionally causes a severe, life-threatening primary pneumonia in normal, healthy children. Viruses probably bring about secondary bacterial pneumonias as often as they cause primary pneumonias. Influenza viruses are notorious in this regard.

The most common bacterial cause of pneumonia is *Streptococcus pneumoniae* (pneumococcus), aptly named for its tendency to infect lung tissue. Usually residing in the throat as part of the normal bacterial flora, this bacterium often takes advantage of viral respiratory infections and gains access to lung tissue. Other bacteria, including group A streptococci and *Staphylococcus aureus*, can also cause secondary pneumonias in this way. *Hemophilus influenzae* type b is a prominent cause of pneumonias in children between 6 and 24 months of age. It is less common in older age groups.

Several categories of organisms other than viruses and bacteria may cause pneumonia. Among them are species of chlamydia and mycoplasma, which share features of both viruses (small size) and bacteria (susceptibility to some antibiotics). There are three species of chlamydia associated with pneumonias. The first, *Chlamydia trachomatis*, is a leading sexually transmitted disease of teens and adults. It also causes pneumonia among young infants during the second and third months of life, producing a mild, progressive illness characterized by persistent, dry cough. This disease is apparently acquired during passage through the birth canal, although symptoms do not appear for several weeks. About half of affected infants have a history of chlamydial eye inflammation (conjunctivitis) during the first weeks of life. A second strain, *Chlamydia psittaci*, may cause psittacosis, a rare respiratory illness usually acquired from pet birds. Finally, *Chlamydia pneumoniae* has been recently discovered to cause pneumonia in older children and adults. *Mycoplasma pneumoniae* also causes pneumonia in older children and adults. Because of the long incubation period and difficulty in making a diagnosis, many epidemics of mycoplasma infections go undetected for weeks or even months after their onset.

Signs and Symptoms

Pneumonia typically begins with an upper respiratory or airways infection. After an interval of apparent improvement, there is a worsening of cough, a recurrence of fever, and a loss of general well-being. Chest pain may occur, especially when the infection causes irritation of the outer lining of the lungs (pleura; pain caused by irritation of the pleura is called pleurisy).

Diagnosis

Pneumonia is suspected in a child or adult who has cough, fever, and characteristic chest noises (audible with a stethoscope). There are three ways of substantiating the diagnosis. The first and most definitive is the chest radiograph, a diagnostic technique that is widely used because it yields important information about the lungs, usually confirming or excluding a diagnosis of pneumonia, lung abscess, or other, less common infectious lung disease. The second diagnostic technique, a culture of sputum, is not useful for children because they cannot usually cough up enough lower respiratory secretions to make a reliable diagnosis. Also less definitive than the chest radiograph, but sometimes helpful nonetheless, are blood tests, including a white cell count and blood culture.

Management

Treatment decisions tend to be based more on the chest radiographic appearance than on the generally less reliable sputum cultures or blood tests. The chest radiograph does not reveal the causative agent, however, so that the child is usually given antibiotics that cover likely and treatable causes. Even though viral pneumonias do not respond to antibiotics, the use of these drugs is acceptable when bacterial agents and *Mycoplasma* species cannot be easily excluded.

Complications

Many pneumonias are themselves complications of preexisting respiratory tract problems. One complication of pneumonia itself is empyema, a collection of pus in the space between the lungs and chest wall. Empyemas may be diagnosed by needle aspiration biopsy and are often drained with a chest tube, which is placed through the skin under local anesthesia.

Recommendations

With respect to contagion, viral pneumonias require no more precautions than the common cold, and only a few bacterial pneumonias are cause for concern. Chief among them is *Hemophilus influenzae* type b pneumonia, which requires the same prophylactic strategy as other invasive diseases caused by this organism (see Chapter 5).

Tuberculosis

Tuberculosis has been a major cause of disease and death throughout human history. Through public health measures and later through antituberculosis drugs, this disease became uncommon in the United States by the 1980s. The 1990s have witnessed both an increase in tuberculosis in the United States and an even more concerning emergence of highly drug-resistant strains. Tuberculosis control has resurfaced as a high public health priority requiring informed and cooperative child care providers.

Tuberculosis is a slowly progressive bacterial infection; it usually affects the lungs but sometimes extends into other organs. Left untreated, tuberculosis can result in serious lung damage and even death.

Cause

Tuberculosis is caused by the organism *Mycobacterium tuberculosis*.

Signs and Symptoms

In the early stages of tuberculosis, the child may be without symptoms. If the disease progresses, fever, fatigue, and weight loss may occur along with dry cough, bloody sputum, and difficulty in breathing. Other symptoms vary with the organs affected.

Diagnosis

The familiar tuberculin skin test is an indicator of exposure to *M tuberculosis*. A positive skin test is followed up with chest radiographs and, sometimes, cultures for the organism to differentiate active tuberculosis from simple exposure.

Management

Treatment for tuberculosis, which lasts for many months, includes rest, good nutrition, and a combination of antituberculous drugs. In unusually severe cases, surgery to remove damaged tissue may be necessary. After the condition has resolved, periodic check-ups should be given for at least 2 years to ensure that the organism does not reactivate.

Complications

Some complications of tuberculosis are more common in young children and include extension of infection into other organ systems, such as the liver, spleen, and brain. Such developments require extended hospitalization and drug therapy.

Recommendations

All cases of tuberculosis should be reported to public health personnel. Skin tests should be given to members of the family and contacts in the school or day care center. Sometimes other children in these settings will have a positive skin test. This almost always indicates exposure to the same adult source because child-to-child contagion is unusual.

Children with positive skin tests usually receive drug therapy (isoniazid) even when the chest radiograph is negative. This is done primarily to prevent reactivation of the organism later in life. Preschool children who have been exposed to adults with known active tuberculosis should receive drug preventive therapy (isoniazid) while awaiting definitive skin test and chest radiograph results. It is likely that broader skin test screening programs will emerge and will include educators and child care providers.

Other Lung Infections

Most lung infections caused by mycobacteria, fungi, and parasites derive their names from the organism itself (eg, histoplasmosis and tuberculosis). These produce chronic, insidious patterns of illness, most com-

Table 10-2 Uncommon Causes of Lower Respiratory Infections

Type of organism	*Disease*	*Causative agent*	*Comments*
Fungi	Histoplasmosis	*Histoplasma capsulatum*	Occurs mostly in midwestern and Ohio River Valley states
	Coccidioidomycosis	*Coccidioides immitis*	Occurs mostly in southwestern states; also called valley fever
	Blastomycosis	*Blastomyces dermatitidis*	Occurs mostly in middle and eastern US
Mycobacteria	Tuberculosis	*Myobacterium tuberculosis*	Still occurs in all regions of US
	Atypical mycobacterial disease	*Myobacterium avium-intracellulare* and others	A major problem in patients with acquired immunodeficiency syndrome
Protozoa	Pneumocystis pneumonia	*Pneumocystis carinii*	Occurs only in immunocompromised persons

monly in restricted geographic areas or in individuals with compromised immunity (Table 10-2).

The usual symptoms of lung infections—fever and relatively unproductive cough—tend to emerge gradually over a period of days or weeks. The chest radiograph may be helpful in diagnosing these conditions.

Most fungal lung diseases, including histoplasmosis and coccidioidomycosis, resolve spontaneously, but the treatment of serious fungal disease and parasitic lung infection tends to be complicated and prolonged, lasting weeks or even months. Children with mycobacterial (other than tuberculosis), fungal, or parasitic lung diseases do not usually pose a threat of contagion to other children.

One other lung disease worthy of mention is lung abscess, a walled-off pocket of pus that usually contains a mixture of bacteria. As a rule, this unusual condition develops only in special circumstances, such as when saliva or vomit is aspirated into the lungs. It is diagnosed with the chest radiograph and special lung tests, and it is treated by drainage and antibiotics.

REFERENCES

Chernick V; Kendig EL, ed. *Kendig's Disorders of the Respiratory Tract in Children.* 5th ed. Philadelphia, Pa: Saunders; 1990.

Cherry JD. Pharyngitis. In: Feigin RD, Cherry JD, eds. *Textbook of Pediatric Infectious Diseases.* 3rd ed. Philadelphia, Pa: Saunders; 1992:159–166.

Moffett HL. *Pediatric Infectious Diseases.* 3rd ed. Philadelphia, Pa: Lippincott; 1989.

Phelan PD, Landau LI, Olinsky A. *Respiratory Illness in Children.* 3rd ed. Oxford: Blackwell Scientific Publications; 1990.

Chapter 11

Gastrointestinal Disease and Hepatitis

GASTROINTESTINAL DISEASE

Inflammation of the gastrointestinal tract (gastroenteritis) is common among young children. The symptoms—vomiting and/or diarrhea sometimes accompanied by nausea and abdominal pain—cause discomfort for the child and worry for parents and caretakers. Most often, vomiting and diarrhea are caused by infectious organisms that are eliminated by the body's natural defense mechanisms. Treatment generally consists of supportive measures such as alterations in diet or increased fluids and, rarely, antimicrobial drugs.

Although vomiting and diarrhea are usually transient and not serious, they sometimes cause dehydration, which can be life threatening, especially in small infants. Vomiting and diarrhea can also signal serious underlying diseases that require prompt diagnosis and treatment.

Vomiting

Vomiting—the forceful evacuation of stomach contents through the mouth, frequently accompanied by nausea—should not be confused with regurgitation (spitting up), which is the loss of all or part of a meal shortly after feeding. Regurgitation is common in infants and usually disappears by 6 to 8 months of age. It is often accompanied by burping but not nausea (an infant who readily feeds after regurgitation is not nauseated).

Rumination, a rare form of chronic regurgitation in infants, can also be confused with vomiting. In this self-stimulating pattern of behavior, the fingers are sucked and mouthed until previously ingested food is regurgitated and then is chewed and swallowed again. Although the exact cause of rumination is unknown, it is sometimes related to psychologic factors, such as poor parent–child interaction. In some cases, there may be abnormal functioning of the esophagus, which causes stomach contents to be regurgitated easily. Treatment addresses both the psychologic and physiologic problems.

Vomiting that begins suddenly is usually caused by infectious organisms (most often viruses) that irritate the stomach or other components of the gastrointestinal tract. Simple cases usually resolve in a day or two. Widespread gastrointestinal illness in the community suggests that a particular child's vomiting is due to this type of infection.

Vomiting is not always due to mild gastrointestinal disorders. It can accompany infections of almost any body organ, including the respiratory tract, the lower intestinal tract, and even the urinary tract (bladder and kidney). Vomiting can also be one of the first recognizable signs of infections of the nervous system (meningitis or encephalitis; see Chapter 9).

Vomiting can signal situations that require emergency medical treatment. One serious condition that is often accompanied by vomiting, especially in young children, is appendicitis. Vomiting can also be a sign of poisoning with cleaning agents, lead, contaminated food or water, toxic gases, and other substances. The drugs used to treat asthma, seizures, heart ailments, and other disorders can cause nausea or vomiting, especially if given or taken in inappropriate doses. An obstructed intestinal tract, seen most commonly in infants, is yet another condition that may be accompanied by vomiting.

Because vomiting can be a sign of life-threatening illnesses, it cannot simply be dismissed as a sign of a mild gastrointestinal disorder until the cause has been investigated, especially with children who are too young to provide verbal clues. As a rule, the younger the child, the more suspicious caretakers must be.

In cases of simple vomiting due to gastroenteritis, food and fluids are generally withheld for a limited time (no longer than 1 hour in the case of an infant). Small sips of clear fluids are gradually reintroduced according to tolerance. A physician should always be consulted in cases of persistent vomiting in which the child is young or does not respond to treatment. Antinausea drugs can be dangerous in young children and are generally not recommended for children of any age.

Because infectious agents that cause vomiting can be readily passed to others, affected children should not return to school or day care until they are able to tolerate food. Alternatively, a child who is vomiting should be isolated from other children with a caretaker who does not care for other children unless they have similar symptoms. Caretakers should wash their hands after contact with affected children and dispose of diapers properly.

Diarrhea

Diarrhea is a messy, unpleasant illness characterized by an increase in the usual frequency, volume, and liquidity of bowel movements (what is usual varies greatly from child to child). As a symptom of gastroenteritis, diarrhea is more common than vomiting. Moreover, it is caused by organisms that present public health problems.

Most cases of diarrhea are due to viral infections of the intestinal tract, which occur principally in the fall, winter, and spring and last between 24 and 48 hours. There may or may not be other symptoms, such as headache, abdominal pain, low-grade fever, malaise, discomfort, or vomiting. Diarrhea that is due to bacteria or other organisms can be more persistent and severe. Infectious diarrhea can become chronic; that is, it can last for more than a few days to a week.

More serious diseases, such as cystic fibrosis or inflammatory bowel disease, can have chronic diarrhea as their initial symptom. Diarrhea can also be a first sign of infections of other body organs (eg, the ears or bladder), especially in young children. Some diarrhea may be due to food intolerances. In some cases, no specific cause for the diarrhea is ever identified. Whatever the cause, diarrhea can be especially serious in infants because it can quickly cause dehydration and upset the chemical balance of body fluids.

With simple diarrhea, tests are not usually done to determine the cause. If symptoms are protracted or unusual, however (eg, blood or mucus in the feces, evidence of dehydration, or high fever), or if the child is young, there is a possibility of serious underlying disease that requires prompt diagnosis. An epidemic of diarrhea in a school or day care setting is another situation in which it may be necessary to determine the cause, and the source, of infection (the public health department can be of considerable help).

When diarrhea-causing organisms are introduced into infant-toddler groups, there is a strong tendency for spread not only within the group but also among child care providers and family contacts. These organisms can be transmitted directly, especially when different groups of children mix freely. The close personal contact and inadequate hygienic practices typical among pre–toilet-trained children provide ready opportunities for spread in day care and preschool groups.

Diarrhea-causing organisms are also spread indirectly by toys and other environmental objects (on which some organisms can survive for up to 6 weeks) and by the hands of caretakers, often through diapering and meal preparation without proper hand washing.

Common Causes of Infectious Diarrhea

Rotavirus. Between 40% and 50% of all diarrhea in infants and young children throughout the world is caused by rotavirus. Rotavirus infection occurs most commonly between the ages of 6 and 24 months, although all age groups are affected. It is most prevalent during the winter.

Diarrhea usually begins from 1 to 3 days after exposure to the rotavirus and may be preceded by vomiting. There is a simple test that detects the rotavirus in stool samples, but this disorder is so common and generally mild that diagnosis is not usually considered necessary. There is no specific treatment, although the physician may recommend dietary changes and increased fluids. No special isolation procedures are required to prevent spread, but good hand washing after diaper changes is important.

Because rotavirus temporarily impairs the intestine's ability to absorb sugar, some children may continue to have diarrhea after the infection has resolved. If the diarrhea lasts more than a few days, however, a physician should be consulted.

Other Viruses. Other viruses besides rotavirus (eg, the Norwalk agent) can cause diarrhea, although they have not been studied as much as rotavirus. The precautions and treatment are the same.

Escherichia coli. The bacterium *Escherichia coli,* although usually a normal intestinal bacterium, can cause diarrhea in several ways. Some strains produce a substance in the intestine that causes fluid to accumulate, producing a watery diarrhea (this strain is typically responsible for traveler's diarrhea). Other strains of *E coli* invade the intestinal lining, causing inflammation and resultant fever, abdominal cramps, and diarrhea that contains mucus and red and white blood cells.

One type of *E coli* has been associated with hemolytic-uremic syndrome (HUS). This syndrome has received national attention in recent years because of outbreaks associated with undercooked meat. Children with HUS experience kidney, blood, and other organ complications with this infection and may have serious, prolonged, or even fatal illness. Sources of *E coli* diarrhea include infected persons, asymptomatic carriers, and food or water that has been contaminated with human feces. This illness is more common in areas with contaminated water supplies or suboptimal sanitation facilities.

The incubation period is from 2 hours to 6 days. Food-borne illness usually occurs within 24 hours of exposure to the bacterium. Treatment depends on the age of the child and the responsible strain of *E coli*. Lost fluids are replaced, usually through oral consumption of electrolyte-containing fluids, and antibiotics are sometimes administered. Affected individuals are contagious as long as they are excreting the organism and should be isolated until the disease has run its course.

Campylobacter *Species*. The bacterium *Campylobacter jejuni* is a common cause of diarrhea in children. It is present in the feces and is transmitted by person-to-person contact or by contaminated food. The illness generally resolves in a few days without treatment, but the organism may be carried, and may infect others, for several weeks after recovery. Symptomatic infected children should be isolated until they have received the antibiotic erythromycin for 5 days.

Salmonella *Species*. Diarrhea caused by the salmonella bacterium occurs primarily in young children, particularly those younger than 1 year. Infection is generally limited to the gastrointestinal tract, but the organism sometimes invades other body tissues, such as blood or bone. Those at risk for the more disseminated illness are young infants, children with sickle cell disease, and children taking drugs that suppress the body's ability to fight infection (eg, drugs to fight cancer or to prevent rejection of organ transplants).

The period between contact with the salmonella organism and the onset of illness (incubation period) is usually less than 24 hours. Treatment consists of oral consumption of electrolyte-containing fluids. Unlike most bacterial diarrhea, that caused by salmonella organisms is not treated with antibiotics (except with children at high risk for spread to other body tissues) because these drugs neither alleviate nor shorten the duration of symptoms and may even prolong the period of communicability.

Because the salmonella organism can be excreted in the feces for weeks or months after symptoms have subsided, affected children should be isolated or cohorted (see Chapter 2) until cultures are negative. Transmission is usually through direct contact with infected persons or contaminated food. Unpasteurized milk is a potential source of infection. Salmonella infection seldom causes outbreaks of diarrhea in day care centers unless there is a common contaminated food source.

One special type of salmonella, *S typhi*, produces a far more serious disease called typhoid fever. Public health departments must be informed when this disease occurs in the community and will make vigorous efforts to track and eradicate it.

Shigella *Species.* Most infections caused by the organism *Shigella sonnei* in this country are mild, consisting only of watery or loose stools for several days. In more severe cases, there can be fever, headache, abdominal cramps, vomiting, urgent diarrhea, or stools containing blood or mucus. A serious form of the disease is bacillary dysentery, in which the child becomes quickly dehydrated as a result of high fever and fluid loss. It is possible to harbor the organism and have no symptoms whatsoever.

Diarrhea caused by Shigella species, like that caused by salmonella organisms, primarily affects children, especially those between 1 and 5 years of age. Outbreaks are common among children in day care centers and institutions and can affect staff and family contacts as well. Only a few organisms are required to cause illness. They are passed in the feces of affected persons. Contaminated food and objects are vehicles of transmission, as are improperly washed hands. Houseflies, too, can transport infected feces.

The incubation period for *Shigella* organisms is usually between 2 and 4 days. Untreated children continue to excrete the organism for several weeks after the symptoms disappear. Antibiotics are given primarily to shorten the time during which the organism is excreted, although they shorten the duration of symptoms as well. Antidiarrheal agents are not recommended for this disorder because they can prolong the course of the disease. Infected children and adults should be isolated until cultures are negative.

Giardia *Species. Giardia* infection is discussed in Chapter 16.

Recommendations

A physician should be notified whenever the affected child is young, when diarrhea lasts more than a few days, or when there are signs of serious illness, such as blood and mucus in the stool, high fever, or dehydration.

The key to preventing the spread of diarrhea-causing organisms is good hand washing with soap and warm water. Staff members should wash their hands upon arrival at work, after diaper changing or helping a child use the toilet, after using the toilet themselves, and before handling food. Children should be taught to wash their hands after toileting and before eating. Regular soap, warm running water, and disposable towels should be made available.

Environmental surfaces, toys, and other objects that children handle or put into their mouths should be cleaned regularly with a disinfectant. A commonly used solution is 1 part chlorine bleach to 10 parts water.

Because diaper changing provides the greatest opportunity for contamination of the child, caretaker, and environment, areas used for this purpose should be designed to facilitate cleaning and hand washing. Diaper areas should be kept physically separate from meal preparation or eating areas and should be disinfected after each diapering. Soiled diapers should be stored in covered containers away from food and materials used by children and staff and out of reach of children. Fecal contents of personal cloth diapers should be emptied into the toilet, and the diapers themselves should be placed in plastic bags, stored in a proper place, and sent home each day with the child.

Whenever possible, groups of children, especially young children, should be physically separated to contain the spread of contagious organisms. Individual staff members should not care for different groups during the day.

A child or staff member with diarrhea is likely to infect others. Segregating children with diarrhea until they can be sent home may reduce the risk of additional cases. During epidemics, it may be necessary to exclude asymptomatic carriers of the organism. Because excluding children creates hardships for parents, especially those who work, large schools or centers may be able to set aside an area where sick children exclusively can be cared for by assigned staff. Alternatively, relatives or volunteer community grandparents may be able to take a sick child during convalescence.

During large outbreaks of diarrhea in schools and day care centers, physicians specializing in infectious diseases should be consulted along with public health officials to help contain the infection and to prevent spread into the community.

HEPATITIS

Hepatitis refers to inflammation of the liver caused by infectious organisms, drugs (eg, overdose of acetaminophen), or toxic substances (eg, carbon tetrachloride, a dry cleaning agent). The more common causes of hepatitis in children are the hepatitis A virus, which is particularly problematic in day care and preschool settings, and the hepatitis B virus.

Hepatitis A

Hepatitis type A is typically a mild illness in children. Its symptoms—fever, diarrhea, or a generally sick feeling—are usually either mild or absent altogether. Only 20% of children younger than 4 years have a serious enough illness to develop jaundice (by contrast, most adults who are infected with hepatitis A develop jaundice).

Affected children, symptomatic and asymptomatic alike, excrete the virus for 1 to 3 weeks in their feces (no other body secretions are likely to transmit the virus). The spread of symptomatic disease among day care personnel, older family members, and other adults in the community may be due in part to transmission among asymptomatic children. The disease is transmitted by direct contact between children, by adults who do not practice good hand washing when handling children or preparing food, and by contaminated environmental objects, on which the virus can remain active for up to 2 weeks.

Epidemics of hepatitis A occur most frequently in day care centers that accept children younger than 2 years, largely because this is the diaper-wearing age (the risk of transmission is much lower among children 4 years old and older). Although affected children have minor, if any, symptoms, adult staff members and parents of center children can become quite ill. Because the period between exposure and the onset of symptoms averages 25 to 30 days, an infection can spread throughout the center before the disease is recognized.

Prevention and control of hepatitis A require strict hygienic standards. This means that day care center staff and parents must be informed about how hepatitis is spread and the importance of proper hand washing, diaper disposal, and toileting procedures. Also important to the control of this disease are early detection before the illness is widespread, reporting cases to public health authorities, and administering immune globulin to exposed persons.

Hepatitis B

Hepatitis B is less common in young children than hepatitis A. Often children do not have symptoms with this disease, although jaundice, loss of appetite, nausea, and a general feeling of weakness are sometimes present. Unlike hepatitis A, hepatitis B can continue to be harbored in the body after the acute infection subsides, posing a risk of chronic infection and, after prolonged carriage, cancer of the liver or cirrhosis.

Hepatitis B is usually transmitted through infected blood products. There is considerably less risk of transmission through saliva and, in contrast to hepatitis A, almost no risk of transmission through feces. The average incubation period is 90 days.

The major concern for school and day care officials is that certain populations can carry infectious hepatitis B particles without being ill themselves. Children who emigrate from endemic areas (such as Korea, Taiwan, and southeast Asian countries) should be screened to determine whether they are carriers of hepatitis B. The health department can furnish updated information about which children should be screened and what precautions should be taken.

Even if a child is identified as being a chronic carrier of the virus, the health hazard to others is minimal. Because the virus is not highly contagious, transmission is not likely to occur to contacts of carrier children under normal hygienic circumstances (routine disinfecting measures destroy the hepatitis B virus). Neither is transmission likely to occur from carriers employed as food handlers or from the use of swimming pools, toilet facilities, or drinking fountains. Nevertheless, care should be taken that the blood of infected individuals or carriers never comes into contact with open wounds of other children or adults. A vaccine is available for susceptible individuals in high-risk work situations, such as hospitals, residential institutions, and school and day care centers that serve populations with a high carriage rate of the hepatitis B virus. The American Academy of Pediatrics now recommends immunization of all infants against hepatitis B.

Hepatitis C

The former term *non-A, non-B hepatitis* has been largely replaced because of newly discovered virus causes. The most prominent of these, discovered in 1989, is called hepatitis C. Most hepatitis C is acquired from blood transfusion.

As many as half the people with hepatitis C will proceed to chronic infection. Some with chronic infection will experience mild or smoldering inflammation of the liver; others will have a more progressive course. Treatment with interferon has reduced liver infection in some individuals.

The risk of transmission of hepatitis C in a child care or school setting has not been formally determined but is believed to be exceedingly low. The much lower rate of mother–infant transmission and of sexual transmission compared with hepatitis B implies that hepatitis C transmission among infants is unlikely to occur. Observation of universal precautions for blood and body fluids should further reduce this hypothetical risk.

REFERENCES

American Academy of Pediatrics. *Report of the Committee on Infectious Diseases*. 22nd ed. Elk Grove Village, Ill: American Academy of Pediatrics; 1991.

American Academy of Pediatrics Committee on Infectious Diseases. Universal hepatitis B immunization. *Amer Acad Pediatr News*. 1992:13–15.

Pickering LK. Bacterial and parasitic enteropathogens in day care. In: Pickering LD, ed. *Infections in Day Care Centers*. Philadelphia, Pa: Saunders, 1990:263–269.

Chapter 12

Genital and Urinary Tract Infections

VULVOVAGINITIS

Vulvovaginitis is characterized by inflammation or irritation of the outer genital area (vulva) and, often, by vaginal discharge. This disorder can result from bacterial, viral, fungal, or parasitic infections as well as from trauma, chemicals, foreign objects, sexual abuse, or allergies.

Cause

Several factors combine to make vaginal infections a relatively common occurrence in prepubertal girls. For one thing, the vagina is an excellent environment for the growth of infectious agents. It is warm and moist and, before adolescence, has a thin protective skin covering. Synthetic panties and tight-fitting clothing help promote irritation and infection by retaining heat and moisture and preventing air circulation. The same is true of disposable diapers with tight-fitting legs and plastic coverings or plastic pants that are worn over cloth diapers.

Another factor that predisposes the vagina to infection is its proximity to the rectum, which makes it vulnerable to bacteria from the intestinal tract. In fact, the organisms most often responsible for vulvovaginitis (such as *Escherichia coli*) are usually those found in the intestinal tract and rectum. Wiping from back to front after a bowel movement can contaminate the vagina with bacteria from the rectum. Shigella organisms, which cause severe gastroenteritis, can also cause vulvovaginitis, even when there is no history of diarrhea. Infection with this organism is characterized by a yellow or green, foul-smelling, and often bloody discharge.

Pinworms (*Enterobius vermicularis*), which commonly infect the gastrointestinal tract of preschool and school-age children, spread to the vagina in 20% of affected girls. These parasites usually cause intense itching of the rectal and vaginal areas, especially at night, when the female worms emerge to lay eggs (see Chapter 16).

Candida albicans, a yeast, can cause vulvovaginitis that is characterized by a beefy red, raised perineal rash with sharp borders surrounded by scattered smaller circular red bumps. There is also a thick, white, cheesy vaginal discharge. Candida vulvitis or vaginitis can result from the spread of candida infections of the diaper area (monilial diaper rash) or mouth (thrush). They can also be contracted from an infected mother during passage through the birth canal. *Candida* vulvitis and vaginitis are more common after antibiotic therapy because antibiotics promote a higher than normal growth of this organism in the intestinal tract. These disorders are also more common in children with diabetes mellitus or immunodeficiencies, who have a lowered resistance to the organism.

The characteristic vesicular or blisterlike lesions of chickenpox can also involve the vulva, resulting in considerable discomfort for the child. The etiology is usually evident in a child with obvious cutaneous manifestations of chickenpox but may be confusing if the first appearance of the rash is in the vulvar area.

Children may also sit in contaminated dirt to play or may touch or scratch the vulvar area with dirty hands. Throat, skin, or respiratory infections can also be spread to the vulva with the hands. One example is the group A streptococcus bacterium (the organism responsible for strep throat and impetigo), which can cause severe vaginitis with a bloody discharge.

Children sometimes insert foreign objects—toys, pieces of food, and most commonly toilet paper—into the vagina during the course of normal exploratory behavior. If these are not removed (usually by a physician), inflammation and infection can occur, often with a persistent, foul-smelling, bloody discharge. Another foreign object that can occasionally be found in the vagina is the clear gel bead used in the construction of superabsorbent disposable diapers. These small compressible beads can sometimes be found in great number on the perineum or discharging from the vagina. These usually cause no symptoms but can be somewhat alarming until the source is identified.

Noninfectious dermatologic conditions can be accompanied by vulvitis. For example, psoriasis and seborrheic or atopic dermatitis, which are usually seen on other areas of the body, can also occur on the vulva. Lichen sclerosis, a rare skin condition, can also cause bleeding of the vulvar area after even minor trauma and is sometimes mistaken for child abuse.

If a child has been abused, sexually transmitted causes of vulvovaginitis such as *Chlamydia trachomatis*, *Trichomonas vaginalis*, and *Neisseria gonorrhoeae* should be considered. Infection with these organisms can cause symptoms ranging from minimal to severe. Although gonorrhea in the young child can occur with no symptoms at all, it is usually accompanied by severe inflammation of the vulva and vagina and a copious, thick, pus-filled discharge. Herpes simplex genital infection can also cause a severe vulvitis or vulvovaginitis in a child or adolescent who has been sexually abused or who is sexually active.

The mucous discharge seen in some newborns is not a sign of vulvovaginitis but a result of stimulation by maternal hormones. By the time the infant is 2 weeks old, these hormones decrease, and occasionally a scant amount of withdrawal bleeding occurs. Although the discharge may be alarming to parents and caretakers, it is of no significance and usually lasts only a few days.

With the exception of withdrawal bleeding in the neonate, vaginal bleeding in a prepubertal child is always significant and should be evaluated by a physician. The cause is most commonly infectious, but other possibilities include trauma (child abuse or accidental or self-inflicted trauma, usually related to scratching), tumor, premature puberty, certain estrogen-containing medications, vaginal foreign body, or structural abnormality of the urethra (urethral prolapse).

Signs and Symptoms

Vulvovaginitis can cause itching, burning, pain with urination, and a discharge that is clear, white, yellow, or green and possibly bloody and foul smelling. The vulva may be red, swollen, and raw. The child may scratch or rub the area, walk awkwardly, and be somewhat irritable. Children with severe infections may avoid urinating as long as possible because of pain when urine comes into contact with the raw vulvar skin.

Labial adhesions, a relatively common finding in young female infants and children, may result as a consequence of vulvovaginitis. These adhesions probably occur when irritation or inflammation of the skin of the vulva causes the labia to adhere or stick together. These adhesions are usually mild, involving only a small part of the labia, and require no therapy. Occasionally the entire labia may be fused, completely obscuring the vaginal opening and causing obstruction of urine flow and poor drainage of vaginal secretions. In this circumstance the physician may prescribe specific treatment, including an estrogen-containing cream, to separate the labia. Forceful separation should not be attempted. This is traumatic for the child and often leads to recurrence of the adhesions.

Diagnosis

The diagnosis of vulvovaginitis is generally made on the basis of characteristic signs and symptoms. Cultures and microscopic examination of the discharge are sometimes necessary to determine the cause of the infection. A physician may also examine the cervix and vagina by using a small instrument inserted into the vagina (vaginoscopy).

Management

Sitz baths in lukewarm water without soap are given from two to four times daily to help clean the affected area and to decrease inflammation and discomfort. The perineum should be patted dry and then allowed to air dry. For children with severe inflammation, premoistened pads (such as Tucks) should be used for wiping rather than toilet paper.

Certain infectious cases of vulvovaginitis, such as those caused by candidal organisms, group A streptococci, and shigella organisms, require specific treatment with a prescribed antibiotic or antifungal agent. If the condition is persistent or recurrent, treatment may include oral or topical antibiotics and/or an estrogen cream applied to the vulvar area to thicken the skin, making it more resistant to infection.

Recommendations

- Children should be taught to wash their hands frequently to prevent the spread of infections.
- Young girls should be instructed to wipe completely from front to back. Because this is more difficult than wiping from the rear forward, careful supervision is necessary. White, unscented toilet tissue decreases the chance of irritation from chemicals.
- White cotton underpants should be used because they are absorbent and allow air circulation. Synthetic panties, tight-fitting clothing, and panty hose should be avoided.
- Harsh, medicated or perfumed soaps and all bubble baths should be avoided.

- For children with sensitive skin who use cloth diapers, an extra rinse in a water and vinegar solution may be needed to remove all soap residues from diapers.
- Diapers of affected children should be changed frequently and left off entirely whenever possible.
- A daily bath, or at least a daily washing of the rectal and genital areas, is desirable for younger children. A mild, nonirritating soap should be used, and the bath should be supervised by a parent.
- Cases of sexually transmitted diseases, such as gonorrhea, in prepubertal children should be reported to local service agencies for investigation of possible sexual abuse.

BALANOPOSTHITIS

Just as young girls may have inflammation of the vulva or vagina, young boys may have inflammation and/or infection of the glans penis and foreskin (balanoposthitis). This condition usually begins as a result of irritation from urine trapped beneath the foreskin and poor hygiene. The inflamed skin then becomes infected, and the foreskin and/or penis may appear swollen and red. The child may complain of tenderness, fever, and pain on urination. Balanoposthitis is usually treated with warm soaks and antibiotics. Circumcision may be recommended for recurrent problems.

URINARY TRACT INFECTIONS

Infections of the urinary tract (Figure 12-1) can involve the bladder (cystitis), the kidney (pyelonephritis), or both. Although urine is normally sterile, urinary tract infections (UTIs), manifested by bacteria in the urine (bacteriuria), are relatively common during childhood. In the neonatal period UTIs are more common in boys. After this time, however, UTIs are much more prevalent among girls. Approximately 1% of boys and 3% of girls have at least one UTI, and as many as 40% of these children have more than one.

Cause

The proximity of the urinary tract to the anus predisposes children to infections of the urinary tract. Approximately 80% to 95% of first UTIs are caused by the bacterium *Escherichia coli,* which is normally found in the intestine. Bacteria from the gastrointestinal tract travel up the urethra to

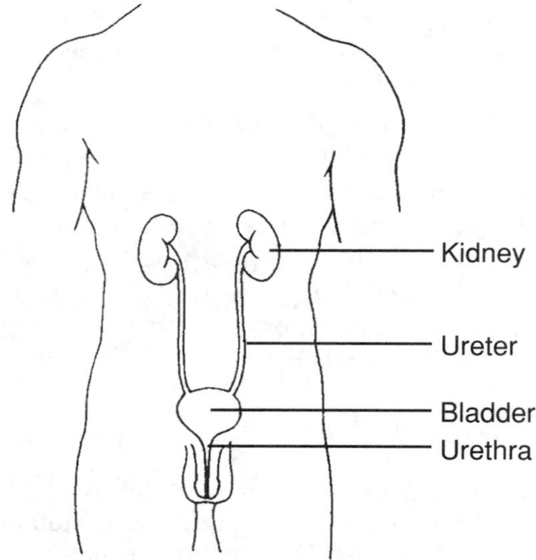

Figure 12-1 The male urinary tract

reach the bladder, where they cause an infection. The fact that the urethra is much shorter in girls than in boys probably accounts for the higher incidence of UTIs among girls.

Certain structural abnormalities of the urinary tract also predispose children to UTIs, particularly those conditions that lead to impaired urine flow or incomplete emptying of the bladder. Also, several recent studies have demonstrated that uncircumcised boys may have a significantly increased risk of UTIs compared with circumcised boys. The reason for this increased risk is not completely known, but experts speculate that the presence of the foreskin may allow bacteria to grow near the area of the urethral opening. These bacteria can cause infection as they ascend through the urethra to the bladder and/or kidneys.

Signs and Symptoms

Signs and symptoms of urinary tract infections can range from mild or absent to severe. In the newborn and young infant, the first signs of infection are usually nonspecific: fever, vomiting, diarrhea, poor feeding, low weight gain, jaundice, listlessness, and irritability. One third of newborns with UTIs have bacteria in their blood stream (bacteremia).

Older infants and children are likely to have symptoms more specific to the urinary system, such as foul-smelling urine, dribbling, pain or burning with urination, increased frequency and urgency of urination, blood in the urine, and bedwetting. Nonspecific symptoms, such as abdominal pain, vomiting, and diarrhea, can also occur. Children with kidney involvement (pyelonephritis) appear particularly ill with high fever, shaking chills, and low back pain.

Diagnosis

The diagnosis of a UTI is based on the result of a urine culture. Urine collection is relatively easy with the toilet-trained child, who simply voids into a sterile container after the genital area has been thoroughly cleansed with soap and water.

Collecting urine from a non–toilet-trained child is more difficult. The usual method involves thoroughly cleansing and drying the entire genital area and then applying a sterile plastic bag that covers the urethra and adheres to the groin. When the child voids, the urine is collected in this bag. Although this collection method causes the least discomfort for the child, it has two major disadvantages: The urine sample can be lost if the bag does not adhere well to the groin, and the urine can become contaminated with bacteria if the genital area has not been properly cleaned or if the bag remains in place for an extended period of time before or after the child voids. For these reasons, many physicians prefer to collect urine samples from infants by inserting a needle into the bladder through the abdomen and withdrawing urine into a syringe (suprapubic aspiration) or by inserting a plastic tube into the bladder through the urethra (catheterization).

In addition to a urine culture, the physician usually performs a urinalysis, checking the urine for blood, sugar, protein, red or white blood cells, and bacteria. If white blood cells (pus cells) and bacteria are present, a UTI is likely. A UTI may be present even if the urinalysis is normal, however.

Management

Although it is possible for some UTIs to resolve spontaneously, antibiotics are given to prevent bacteremia (bacteria in the blood stream) or kidney involvement with subsequent scarring and decreased kidney function. Children are usually treated for 10 to 14 days with oral doses of either a penicillin (such as amoxicillin), a sulfonamide, a trimethoprim-sulfamethoxazole combination, or a cephalosporin. If the child is young or appears to be very sick with high fever or shaking chills, hospitalization and intravenous antibiotics may be recommended.

Follow-up urine cultures should be performed frequently during the first year after a UTI because the disease can recur without symptoms. After a documented UTI, boys of any age and girls younger than approximately 5 years are usually evaluated by X-ray studies and/or ultrasound for abnormalities of the urinary tract. Girls older than 5 years at the time of their first UTI generally do not need this kind of evaluation unless they have a recurrence of infection or other evidence of kidney abnormality or dysfunction, such as poor growth, high blood pressure, or abnormalities of the genitals.

Radiologic evaluation after a UTI usually includes renal (kidney) ultrasound and a voiding cystourethrogram (VCUG), which determines how well the bladder empties and whether there is abnormal flow of urine from the bladder to the kidneys (reflux). During a VCUG, a catheter inserted through the urethra injects dye into the bladder, and radiographs are obtained as the child voids. If the VCUG is abnormal, evaluation may also include further studies of the kidney.

The aim of radiologic evaluation is to detect any abnormality that may predispose the child to reinfection and/or progressive kidney damage. Some such abnormalities require surgical correction; others require only long-term use of low-dose antibiotics to prevent reinfection.

Children with certain conditions (eg, meningomyelocele, also called spina bifida) are particularly prone to UTIs and may require intermittent bladder catheterization to avoid infection. At times it may be necessary to call upon school personnel to assist with this simple but important procedure. In addition, some experts recommend circumcision for young male infants with a proven UTI in the first several months of life.

Complications

Complications associated with UTIs include progression of the infection to involve the blood stream (bacteremia) or kidneys. Involvement of the kidneys can cause scarring with subsequent loss of function. In extreme cases, complete kidney failure can occur. When this happens, a kidney transplant and/or dialysis may be necessary.

Recommendations

Good hygiene is important in preventing UTIs. Girls should be taught always to wipe from front to back after a bowel movement to avoid contaminating the urethral area.

Urinary tract infections are not contagious and do not require exclusion from school or day care.

Any of the following symptoms should be reported to parents:

- burning or pain upon urination
- increased frequency of urination
- bedwetting in a child who was previously dry during naps or at night
- urine that is foul smelling or contains blood

REFERENCES

Altchek A. Recognizing and controlling vulvovaginitis in children. *Contemp Pediatr*. 1985; 2: 59–70.

Emans SJ. Vulvovaginitis in the child and adolescent. *Pediatr Rev*. 1986; 8:12–19.

Feld LG, Greenfield SP, Ogra PL. Urinary tract infections in infants and children. *Pediatr Rev*. 1989; 2:71–77.

Hansson S, Jodal U, Noren L, Bjure J. Untreated bacteriuria in asymptomatic girls with renal scarring. *Pediatrics*. 1989; 84:964–968.

Wald ER. Gynecologic infections in the pediatric age group. *Pediatr Infect Dis*. 1984; 3:S10–S13.

Williams TS, Callen JP, Owen LG. Vulvar disorders in the prepubertal female. *Pediatr Ann*. 1986; 15:588–605.

Wiswell TE, Enzenauer RW, Holton ME, Cornish JD, Hankins CT. Declining frequency of circumcision: implications for changes in the absolute incidence and male to female sex ratio of urinary tract infections in early infancy. *Pediatrics*. 1987; 79:338–342.

Chapter 13

Rashes and Skin Infections

Skin rashes accompany a seemingly infinite number of human diseases, infectious and noninfectious alike (Table 13-1). The appearance and distribution of the rash is usually distinctive enough to permit prompt diagnosis. At times, however, certain noninfectious rashes (eg, drug reactions) can mimic those caused by infectious diseases. Moreover, the same organism can cause one kind of rash by a direct skin infection and another kind of rash when the infection is elsewhere in the body. Group A streptococci, for example, cause both the crusted sores of impetigo and the bright red rash that accompanies scarlet fever.

CHICKENPOX

Chickenpox (varicella) is one of two different diseases (the other is shingles) caused by the varicella-zoster virus. *Chickenpox* is the term used for the initial infection with the virus, in which a generalized rash appears on many parts of the body (see Color Plate 4, a and b). Chickenpox is exceedingly common in this country, as evidenced by the prevalence of serum antibodies (signs of a previous encounter with the virus) in American adults. The fact that many of these people do not remember having childhood chickenpox probably means that the rash was mild enough to go unnoticed. Generally speaking, however, rash is the most prominent feature of chickenpox and typically appears in crops of vesicles. (These tiny, fluid-filled lesions with a red base have been described as dew drops on rose petals).

The rash, usually more prominent on the trunk and abdomen than on the extremities, often causes substantial itching, which can interrupt sleep and lead to secondary bacterial infection from scratching. Other common symptoms of chickenpox are fever, malaise, and headache. All these symptoms usually disappear within 5 to 7 days.

Table 13-1 Common Infection-Related Rashes of Children

Infecting agent	*Disease*	*Comments*
Viral	Chickenpox (varicella) Shingles (zoster)	Caused by the same virus. Vaccine and antiviral therapy are changing clinical strategy.
	Measles Rubella	Immunization has made both rare in the US.
	Erythema infectiosum Roseola	Also called "fifth disease". Rash at end of illness.
	Warts Molluscum contagiosum	May be present for prolonged period.
Rickettsial	Rocky Mountain spotted fever	Most common in eastern and southern US. Early diagnosis is crucial.
Bacterial	Impetigo Cellulitis	Usually caused by group A streptococci. Can be caused by various bacteria.

Chickenpox is one of the most contagious of all childhood illnesses. Affected children should be isolated from nonimmune children and adults until all lesions are crusted over. Although skin lesions contain infectious particles, they are not the main source of contagion. The usual mode of transmission is actually respiratory. It happens that respiratory excretion of the virus ceases at about the same time that all the lesions are crusted over.

Chickenpox is diagnosed more often by parents or grandparents than by physicians, largely because the accompanying rash is so distinctive. In situations where medical attention is sought, the diagnosis is also usually made by visual inspection. With certain individuals, however, such as newborns, pregnant women, or cancer patients, more definitive diagnostic procedures are necessary.

Treatment for chickenpox depends entirely upon the age and health status of the host. Children usually require little more than lotions to control itching and acetaminophen for fever. Aspirin should be avoided because of its link with Reye syndrome (see Chapter 17).

When there is risk of severe disease, the antiviral agent acyclovir is also given, usually intravenously (which requires hospitalization). An oral form of this medication is available as well and has been used in normal children. Most experts believe that the severity of chickenpox in older adolescents and adults is sufficient to justify oral acyclovir use. The modest benefit of this drug and the more benign course of disease in young children have led most practitioners not to treat routinely unless there are questions of immune status. There is considerable variation among physicians in this realm.

Complications of chickenpox, although uncommon, can be serious. In rare cases, children with chickenpox develop Reye syndrome, or hemorrhaging of blood vessels in the skin or other organs (hemorrhagic varicella). Chickenpox is generally less severe in children than adults, however, who frequently develop pneumonia. Pregnant women can have unusually severe illness, and in rare cases the virus infects the fetus. Newborns whose mothers develop chickenpox within several days of delivery are at risk for serious or fatal disease, such as infection of the liver and lungs, although this can usually be prevented with a special γ globulin. Similarly, children with impaired immunity (eg, those receiving cancer chemotherapy or steroid medication) are at risk for severe, and likewise preventable, chickenpox infection. Perhaps the most common complication of chickenpox is secondary bacterial infection—often by *Staphylococcus aureus* or a Group A streptococcus—of the skin lesions. This infection may be treated with topical or oral antibiotics or, in severe cases, intravenous antibiotics.

A live but attenuated vaccine against the varicella zoster virus has been developed, and approval is pending. It is likely that if and when the vaccine is approved it will be incorporated into the routine immunization sequence, perhaps with the measles, mumps, and rubella vaccine.

Children with chickenpox should be excluded from school or child care until all lesions are crusted over. The period of presumed contagion extends from 1 or 2 days before the onset of symptoms to approximately 1 week afterward. Children with compromised immune systems who are exposed to chickenpox should be seen promptly by a physician. Care providers who have not had chickenpox should consult a physician if they are exposed to this disease. Chickenpox may be unusually severe in adults. Pregnant women who are not immune to chickenpox should avoid contact with affected children and should seek medical attention promptly if exposure or symptoms occur.

SHINGLES

Shingles (zoster, sometimes called herpes zoster because the characteristic skin lesions, when viewed under a microscope, resemble the lesions caused by herpes simplex virus) is a rash caused by reactivation of the varicella-zoster virus in a person who has had chickenpox (varicella). In contrast to the generalized rash of chickenpox, shingles consists of a localized band of vesicles that does not generally cross the midline of the body (see Color Plate 5). These vesicles are often painful and are sometimes accompanied by fever or swollen lymph nodes in the area.

The interval between chickenpox and shingles may be years or even decades. It is believed that the varicella-zoster virus, like herpes simplex virus, resides in a hidden (latent) state in the body between recurrences. This disease is more common in the elderly, possibly because of the weakening of the immune system later in life.

Shingles is distinctly uncommon during childhood, occurring primarily in children who had chickenpox before or soon after birth and in children with impaired immunity who had chickenpox previously.

The diagnosis of shingles is usually made by simple visual inspection of the lesions. Their unique distribution and vesicular character usually make other diagnostic tests unnecessary. As with chickenpox, however, scrapings of the skin lesions (the Tzanck preparation) are sometimes viewed under a microscope. If these reveal characteristic multinucleated giant cells, the possible causes for the lesions are narrowed down to herpes simplex and varicella-zoster viruses. A culture can then be obtained to distinguish between these two agents.

Management for shingles, like that for chickenpox, depends on the immune status of the child. In adults (and presumably children) with impaired immunity, the antiviral agent acyclovir helps speed recovery. This drug may also benefit normal children with zoster.

The most annoying complication of shingles is prolonged pain in the rash area after the vesicles have disappeared (postherpetic neuralgia). This sometimes incapacitating sequela to zoster is common in adults and may be amenable to steroids in the elderly. Children rarely experience this kind of pain.

Another complication of shingles, seen almost exclusively in immunologically compromised children and adults, is extension of the lesions well beyond the localized band to other parts of the skin and even to internal organs. Treatment for disseminated shingles is intravenous antiviral therapy.

Unlike chickenpox, shingles is characterized by little or no respiratory excretion of the virus. Even so, contagion is possible through direct contact with lesions that are not yet crusted over. Children or adults with shingles can prevent transmission by covering affected areas.

Although shingles is far less contagious than chickenpox, the varicella-zoster virus is still a potential threat to children with impaired immunity. Direct physical contact between children with shingles and immunologically impaired children who have not already had chickenpox should be avoided; if such contact occurs, a physician should be notified.

MEASLES

Measles (rubeola), an illness caused by the measles virus, is characterized initially by fever, cough, and inflammation of the conjunctivae (conjunctivitis) and upper respiratory tract. These manifestations are followed within several days by a distinctive and florid rash, which often persists for a week (see Color Plate 6, a and b). This generalized rash is more prominent on the face and upper body and becomes confluent by the third or fourth day after its appearance.

Diagnosis of measles is made by visually inspecting the rash, culturing the virus from the throat, and studying serum for an increase in antibodies to the virus. Management of fever is generally all the treatment that is required unless there are complications, such as pneumonia or inflammation of the brain (encephalitis). Encephalitis, which occurs in about 1 in every 1,000 measles cases, was a primary impetus for vaccine development.

Vaccines for measles have been in use since the 1960s. Children in the United States now receive measles immunization, usually along with mumps and rubella vaccines, at 15 months of age. Because of the inadequacy of certain early vaccines, some individuals may still be susceptible to measles. Several colleges experienced measles outbreaks in the early 1980s, and many have responded with measles immunization programs for students. Community outbreaks have occurred in the 1990s and reflect both the underimmunization of urban populations and the waning of immunity after a single vaccine. It is now recommended that children receive two measles, mumps, and rubella vaccines during childhood to ensure adequate immunity (see Chapter 3 on immunizations). Measles is a highly contagious disease; although it is now rare in the United States, it remains a serious problem in developing countries, where it frequently causes death in malnourished infants.

If a case of measles (or suspected measles) occurs, affected individuals should be isolated and public health officials notified at once.

RUBELLA

Rubella (also called German measles and 3-day measles) is a relatively brief infectious illness, usually involving several days of malaise and lymph node enlargement followed by a 3-day course of rash, fever, and inflamed conjunctivae and throat. As with measles, the rubella rash is more prominent on the face and upper body, but the rubella rash is more subtle, and the lesions are usually not confluent. Fever and other symptoms are also considerably milder than with measles.

Rubella is a mild disease that rarely causes complications in children, but it can have devastating effects on an unborn fetus when a nonimmune woman is infected during the first trimester of pregnancy (see Chapter 14).

As with measles, the diagnosis of rubella is usually made by visually inspecting the rash, culturing the rubella virus from the throat, and examining serum for increases in antibodies to the virus. A blood test for these antibodies is performed on all pregnant women and on most children with congenital infection from an unknown cause. Children and adults with rubella are treated with antifever medications.

Although major outbreaks of rubella have not occurred in the United States since 1969, sporadic cases continue to be reported. Since 1988, in fact, the incidence of rubella has risen dramatically, with more than 1,000 cases being reported in 1990. There has been a simultaneous rise in reports of the congenital rubella syndrome during this time.

All children or adults with rubella or suspected rubella should be isolated from other individuals. In particular, nonimmune pregnant women should avoid contact with persons with rubella. Although mass immunization has made outbreaks unlikely, there is increasing concern that a sizable number of young women in their childbearing years remain nonimmune. Therefore, each case of rubella has substantial implications for public health. Public health officials should be notified promptly of any suspected or identified cases.

ERYTHEMA INFECTIOSUM

Erythema infectiosum (also known as fifth disease because it was fifth on an old listing of rashes in children) is a mild skin disorder. It is characterized by a slapped-cheek redness of the face that is followed by a generalized rash that appears most prominently on the extremities and extends to other parts of the body. There may also be a slight fever.

A contagious disease, erythema infectiosum is common in the United States, often occurring in epidemics among young children. The incubation period appears to be 1 or 2 weeks. In addition to the mild childhood disease, arthritis may develop in adults when they encounter this agent. More important, infection with this agent during pregnancy apparently poses risk of fetal injury or loss (discussed in detail in Chapter 6). The causal agent, discovered in the 1980s, is parvovirus B19.

Diagnosis in childhood rests on visual inspection. The classic slapped-check face or a known epidemic of erythema infectiosum in the community is a helpful indicator. If fever is present, antifever medications may be given, but no other treatment is necessary. Occasionally, the rash recurs after days or weeks, but it promptly subsides.

Children with erythema infectiosum pose no threat of severe disease to their classmates. This is apparently true even of classmates who have impaired immunity. Affected children need not be excluded from child care or school after diagnosis (even if rash is present) because children are unlikely to be contagious after the rash has become manifest. Women who are pregnant or anticipating pregnancy should follow precautions outlined in Chapter 6 to minimize risk of acquiring this virus during pregnancy.

ROSEOLA

Roseola (exanthema subitum, sometimes called roseola infantum) is an early childhood illness characterized by approximately 4 days of high fever followed by a generalized rash. This disease can occur at any time of the year and primarily affects preschool children, most commonly those between 6 and 24 months of age. The concentration of roseola in this age group may reflect the ubiquitous character of the virus or the lack of symptoms in older age groups. The virus that causes roseola was discovered in 1988 and has been termed human herpesvirus 6.

Diagnosis of roseola before the fourth day is difficult. In most cases, the only sign or symptom present during the first few days is fever (although occasionally there is also inflammation of the throat or conjunctivae and mild swelling of the lymph nodes). The most helpful diagnostic feature is the classic rash: discrete red spots, especially on the trunk and neck, that usually appear precisely at the time the fever subsides.

Once it is determined that the high fever is due to roseola and not some other disorder, treatment is generally limited to antifever medications. Complications of roseola are uncommon, although the abrupt onset and magnitude of fever can cause febrile convulsions in children who are predisposed (see Chapter 4). It appears that human herpesvirus 6 may be an uncommon cause of neurologic infection in other age groups as well as infants.

Roseola is probably communicable during the period of acute febrile illness, although the degree of this communicability is unknown. The risk to other children appears to be minimal, but it is prudent to exclude affected children from contact with other children during the period of fever and acute illness.

WARTS

Warts are easily recognizable bumps with a hard texture caused by increased production of a skin protein (keratin) in response to certain papovaviruses (see Color Plate 7).

Person-to-person transmission is assumed, although it is rarely possible to identify a source or to recognize group outbreaks. Warts occur in all ages and on many parts of the body. Skin specialists divide them into four categories: flat warts, common warts, plantar warts, and venereal warts. Flat warts are less prominently raised than other warts and occur primarily on the face and hands of children. Common warts are raised warts found most frequently on the hands; they occur in all ages. Plantar warts, so called because they occur on the plantar surface (soles) of the foot, are less of a cosmetic problem than other warts, but they can cause pain on walking. Venereal warts occur in the genital or anal area and are transmitted sexually.

Warts are diagnosed by visual inspection. Treatment usually consists of ointments, soaks, mechanical paring of the lesion, or freezing with liquid nitrogen. Most warts disappear spontaneously, although they may last for months or even years.

Complications of warts are uncommon. Venereal warts in a pregnant woman can cause warts in the larynx of the infant (laryngeal papillomatosis) unless the child is delivered by cesarean section. Other complications can arise as consequences of therapy (eg, aggressive paring or irritating ointments and soaks).

Nonvenereal warts are neither very contagious nor very serious, and their prolonged duration makes efforts at preventing spread impractical. Warts near a child's genitals or anus may be sexually transmitted, suggesting sexual abuse. They should be reported to a physician.

MOLLUSCUM CONTAGIOSUM

Molluscum contagiosum, a skin infection commonly found in children and young adults, consists of small, waxy-appearing bumps with dimpling (umbilicated papules) at the center. In children, this rash may appear anywhere on the face, trunk, or extremities and is believed to be transmitted by direct contact with the lesions. Children with eczema (atopic dermatitis) appear to be at increased risk for acquiring this disorder. By adulthood, molluscum contagiosum is usually found in the genital or anal region and is transmitted sexually.

Molluscum contagiosum is caused by a member of the poxvirus group. Although epidemics have been reported among young children in situations such as boarding schools, the source of infection is usually unknown.

Because the responsible virus cannot be cultured, diagnosis of this skin disorder is based on visual inspection. Treatment usually consists of simple removal with a looplike instrument (curette) followed by application of various topical compounds. Like warts, molluscum contagiosum usually resolves spontaneously, but it may last for months or even years.

As with warts, the low infectivity, mild nature, and extended duration of molluscum contagiosum make most efforts at preventing transmission impractical.

SMALLPOX

Smallpox is a serious, often fatal disease characterized by a distinctive rash and fever. In 1980, the World Health Organization announced that its global campaign to eradicate smallpox had been successful. Today, the smallpox virus exists only in four special laboratories and no longer poses a threat to human health. This magnificent accomplishment offers hope that through concerted effort and international cooperation other infectious diseases can also be completely eradicated.

NONSPECIFIC VIRAL RASH

The term *nonspecific viral rash* is often applied, albeit reluctantly, to nondescript or faint rashes that accompany viral diseases of undetermined nature, particularly among children. Certain viruses, such as enteroviruses, produce many different kinds of rashes, making them likely causes of unidentified rashes.

ROCKY MOUNTAIN SPOTTED FEVER

Rocky Mountain spotted fever is a potentially fatal disease characterized by a distinctive rash and fever. Despite its name, this disorder occurs most commonly in the eastern and southern states. It is caused by a rickettsia (*Rickettsia rickettsii*), that is carried by hard ticks (*Ixodes* species).

Symptoms (fever, headache, muscle aches, and chills) appear between 4 days and 2 weeks after the tick bite. Then, within 2 to 4 days after the onset of fever, a distinct spotted rash appears all over the body, including the palms and soles.

Diagnosis of Rocky Mountain spotted fever is suggested by the characteristic rash; this rash may not appear for up to 5 days after the onset of illness, however. Study of a skin biopsy specimen under a microscope can reveal the organism, but this procedure is not widely available. Blood studies can confirm the diagnosis, but they take time. Consequently, treatment usually begins with a presumptive rather than a definitive diagnosis.

Management consists of antibiotics and close observation for complications, such as inflammation of the brain (encephalitis) and hemorrhaging of small blood vessels throughout the body. In areas where Rocky Mountain spotted fever is common, children with mild illness may be treated outside the hospital.

Children or adults with suspected Rocky Mountain spotted fever should be seen by a physician promptly for appropriate diagnostic testing. Because person-to-person transmission is not known to occur, affected children can return to the child care or classroom setting as soon as they feel well enough to do so. Precautions for contacts are unnecessary.

IMPETIGO

Impetigo is a bacterial skin infection that often begins around the nose and mouth (see Color Plate 8). The characteristic lesions, usually covered with a brownish-yellow crust, typically appear at the site of minor trauma and then spread to normal skin nearby. The infection can be spread to other parts of the body as well, usually by the hands.

Impetigo is common among children and often spreads in families, schools, or neighborhoods through contact with the infected area. It is typically caused by group A streptococci bacteria. At times *Staphylococcus aureus* is found in the lesions as well, in which case they may have a blistery appearance (bullous impetigo).

Diagnosis is generally based on visual inspection, although a culture of the lesions usually reveals the responsible agent. Treatment generally consists of injected or oral penicillin and, at times, topical antibacterial ointments.

Impetigo itself is not a serious disorder, but it occasionally results in acute poststreptococcal glomerulonephritis, an inflammatory condition affecting the kidneys. Interestingly, the strains of group A streptococci that produce impetigo are not associated with rheumatic fever, the other major complication of strep throat (see Chapter 10).

Children with impetigo (like children with strep throat) should be treated with antibiotics and allowed to return to child care or school after 24 hours of antibiotic therapy. In extensive outbreaks, groups of children are sometimes given prophylactic penicillin to prevent further spread. Such efforts should be coordinated by health officials.

CELLULITIS

Cellulitis is a localized infection of the tissue just beneath the skin causing swelling and pain of this tissue along with reddish or bluish discoloration of the skin itself. This disorder commonly occurs around the eyes and on the cheeks, buttocks, and extremities.

Cellulitis can be caused by a number of bacteria, particularly *Staphylococcus aureus*, group A streptococci, and *Hemophilus influenzae* type b. If the cellulitis occurs after bites or other trauma, the responsible bacteria may be related to the source (eg, *Pasteurella multocida* from a dog's mouth). The location and color of the cellulitis, the age of the child, and the presence or absence of preceding trauma are all important clues in determining the responsible bacteria.

Symptoms of cellulitis typically include swelling, tenderness, discoloration of the skin, and sometimes fever. Some symptoms are specific to the area involved. For example, cellulitis in the cavity behind the eye (orbital cellulitis) disturbs vision and causes pain with eye movement. This is not true of cellulitis in the soft tissue around but not behind the eye (preseptal or periorbital cellulitis).

Diagnosis begins with an inspection of the affected area to determine which cultures are appropriate. Bacteria for some cultures are obtained by needle aspiration, although this technique is not routinely used around the eye. Blood culture, especially in the young child with fever, may also be helpful.

Management for serious cellulitis consists of hospitalization with intravenous antibiotics. Often with orbital cellulitis, pus must be surgically drained from the space behind the eye. Other types of cellulitis may benefit from warm compresses applied over the skin. Once the infection is under control, antibiotics are often given orally, making further hospitalization unnecessary.

Complications of cellulitis depend on the causative organism and the site of infection. If the infection is near the eye, for example, damage to vision may result. Occasionally the bacteria travel through the blood stream to other areas of the body, causing infection of the central nervous system (meningitis) or joints (septic arthritis). This complication is most common in preschool children with untreated cellulitis caused by *H influenzae* type b.

Most of the bacteria that cause cellulitis are not very contagious. Each bacterial agent has particular implications, however. For example, group A streptococci have little contagious potential after 48 hours of appropriate antibiotic therapy, and *Staphylococcus aureus*, which usually enters breaks in the skin at the time of the inciting trauma, does not spread to other children. *Hemophilus influenzae* type b has more important implications (see Chapter 5).

Cellulitis that follows an animal bite may bring a child to medical attention for the first time since the bite. If so, questions regarding the status of the animal's rabies immunization and the child's tetanus immunization must also be addressed.

DIAPER RASHES

The dampness of the diaper area inevitably promotes irritation and growth of microorganisms, making diaper rashes one of the most common rashes of early childhood. The initial cause of most diaper rash is the irritating effect of the ammonia in urine, although feces and chemical agents can also cause irritation. Often, this rash becomes infected with bacteria or yeast, producing more distinctive lesions (see Color Plate 9).

Diagnosis is usually made by visual inspection. If secondary infection is suspected, however, the rash can be scraped and the organism cultured for identification under a microscope. Healing is usually facilitated by keeping the area as dry as possible. It may be necessary to leave the area open to air or to avoid occlusive pants over the diapers. Topical ointments such as zinc oxide, cortisonelike drugs, antibiotics, or antifungal agents may be applied to the diaper area (which ointment is used depends on the suspected cause).

Approaches to treating diaper rashes vary widely, depending on the responsible agent and parental and physician preference. Perhaps the only overriding principle of treatment is that frequent diaper changes reduce the likelihood that an existing rash will be exacerbated.

REFERENCES

Dobson RL, Abele DC. *The Practice of Dermatology*. Philadelphia, Pa: Harper & Row; 1985.

Goodman T. *The Skin Doctor's Skin Doctoring Book*. New York, NY: Sterling; 1984.

Hurwitz S. *Clinical Pediatric Dermatology*. 2nd ed. Philadelphia, Pa: Saunders; 1993.

Krugman S, Katz SL, Gershon AA, Wilfert CM. *Infectious Diseases of Children*. St Louis, Mo: Mosby; 1992.

Chapter 14

Cytomegalovirus, Herpes, and Other Congenital Infections

Despite immunization programs and effective antimicrobial medications for many infectious agents, congenital infections (ie, infections that occur before birth) remain an important cause of birth defects among children throughout the world. Because the agents responsible for these infections can damage the brain, eyes, or ears along with other body organs, survivors often have long-term disabilities that influence motor and intellectual performance.

Relatively few infectious agents can cause congenital infections (Exhibit 14-1). These agents—viruses, spirochetes, and protozoa—tend to produce similar signs and symptoms and have been categorized historically as the TORCH or STORCH syndrome. The letters of the latter acronym stand for syphilis, toxoplasmosis, other organisms, rubella, cytomegalovirus (CMV), and herpes.

Most STORCH agents are acquired during close contact with other humans. Certain agents are present in the body secretions (eg, saliva or urine) or blood of infected persons and are transmitted by direct exposure to the infected body fluid. Some STORCH agents, including syphilis, herpes simplex viruses (HSVs), and CMV, may be present in cervical secretions or semen and can be transmitted sexually.

Although women may have many different illnesses during pregnancy (such as colds, flu, or gastrointestinal disorders), these rarely result in serious fetal infections. If the infection is with a STORCH agent, however, there is a risk of fetal death, miscarriage, or birth defect. If the mother is immune to the particular agent (eg, through vaccination or prior exposure), the fetus will not be seriously affected. If the mother is not immune,

Exhibit 14-1 Agents That Cause Congenital Infections

Viruses	*Spirochetes*
CMV	*Treponema pallidum* (syphilis)
HSVs	*Borrelia burgdorferi* (Lyme disease)
Rubella virus	
Varicella zoster virus	*Protozoa*
Human immunodeficiency virus	*Toxoplasma gondii*
Enteroviruses	*Trypanosoma cruzi* (Chagas' disease)
Lymphocytic choriomeningitis virus	*Plasmodium* species (malaria)

however, the agent can be carried by the blood stream to the placenta, and the fetus may become infected.

A STORCH agent can affect the fetus by damaging the placenta (which alters the blood supply to the fetus) or by directly injuring the developing fetal organs. The extent of the damage depends upon the infectious agent and the stage of pregnancy at which infection occurs. Infections acquired early in pregnancy tend to result in more serious birth defects, whereas infections later in pregnancy may produce no visible signs of damage.

Congenital infections can cause numerous long-term abnormalities. Most of the abnormalities listed in Exhibit 14-2 can be caused by any one of the infectious agents described in this chapter. Some agents produce specific abnormalities, however. Congenital heart defects are usually associated with rubella (German measles), and scarring of the skin can be caused by herpes, chickenpox (varicella zoster virus), and syphilis.

The most serious consequences of congenital infections are the damaging effects on the brain, eyes, and ears. As a result, infected infants may have shortened life spans or long-term intellectual and perceptual disabilities. Although many of these children can eventually enter regular educational or child care environments, others are so severely affected that they require long-term specialized care.

SYPHILIS

Syphilis, an infection with the spirochete *Treponema pallidum,* remains an important health problem throughout the world. Beginning in the 1980s, cases of syphilis among women of childbearing age in the United States rose substantially, leading to a dramatic increase in the numbers of infants with congenital syphilis. This increase reflected several factors, in-

Exhibit 14-2 Complications of Congenital Infections

Fetal death and miscarriage Stillbirth Shortened life span Seizures Developmental or mental retardation Blindness (cataracts, chorioretinitis, optic nerve abnormalities) Deafness Deficient brain growth (microcephaly) Hydrocephalus Congenital heart defects Abnormal muscle tone Poor body growth Abnormal bones or teeth Glandular disturbances (thyroid dysfunction, diabetes mellitus)

cluding prostitution, drug use, acquired immunodeficiency syndrome (AIDS), limited access to medical care, and a modified definition of congenital syphilis. Currently, more than 3,000 infants with congenital syphilis are born annually in the United States alone.

Syphilis is typically transmitted by sexual contact with an infected individual. The signs and symptoms of syphilis in adults depend, in part, on how long an individual has been infected. Primary (or early) syphilis, the most common form, is a localized lesion, or chancre, at the site of initial infection. In secondary syphilis, the disease is extended to the skin, the membranes of the mouth and genitals, and other organs and tissues. Tertiary (or late) syphilis can involve nearly any organ system.

Congenital syphilis occurs when the treponemal organisms invade the mother's blood stream and are carried to the placenta. The risk of congenital syphilis is greatest during the primary or secondary stages of the disease, when more than 70% of untreated mothers transmit infection to their unborn infants. Many infected fetuses die, resulting in a miscarriage.

Infants born with congenital syphilis have signs of multiple organ involvement (Table 14-1), and some untreated infants may die within a few months. Untreated survivors manifest signs of congenital syphilis later in life, including abnormal teeth, nerve deafness, scarring of the skin and lips, bony abnormalities, inflammation of the cornea and conjunctiva, and mental retardation.

A diagnosis of syphilis is established by testing the blood of both mother and infant for antibodies to the treponemal organisms. The two

Table 14-1 Common Features of Congenital Infection

Feature	*Syphilis*	*Toxoplasmosis*	*Rubella*	*CMV*	*HSV*
Liver/spleen enlargement	+	+	+	+	+
Low birth weight	+	+	+	+	+
Anemia	+	+	+	+	+
Low platelet count	+	+	+	+	+
Jaundice	+	+	+	+	+
Small head size	+	+	+	+	+
Eye abnormalities	+	+	+	+	+
Brain calcifications		+	+	+	+
Seizures	+	+	+	+	+
Hydrocephalus	+	+		+	+
Bone abnormalities	+		+		
Congenital heart defects			+		
Skin rash	+	+	+	+	+

most commonly used tests are the Venereal Disease Research Laboratory test and the fluorescent treponemal antigen test. Both are routinely available through most hospitals and health departments.

Congenital syphilis can be prevented by treating the infected mother with the antibiotic penicillin. All pregnant women should have a serologic test for syphilis early in pregnancy and again during the last trimester. Treatment recommendations can be obtained from physicians or local health departments.

Infants who are born with congenital syphilis should also be treated with penicillin to prevent later complications. Current strategies for treatment of congenital syphilis can be found in the *Red Book*, published by the Committee on Infectious Diseases of the American Academy of Pediatrics (141 Northwest Point Boulevard, PO Box 927, Elk Grove Village, IL 60009-0927). Treated infants pose no risk to exposed individuals, but until treatment is completed, these infants should be excluded from day care programs.

TOXOPLASMOSIS

Toxoplasmosis, caused by infection with the protozoan *Toxoplasma gondii*, is the second most common human congenital infection, affecting as many as 1 in every 1,000 live births in the United States. Rates of toxoplasmosis vary throughout the world and depend on age, geographic location, and dietary practices. In the United States, approximately 3,000 children with congenital toxoplasmosis are born annually.

Unlike most other organisms that cause congenital infections, *T gondii* is acquired from nonhuman sources. This parasite uses cats as its primary host but can infect many different species of birds and mammals. Humans become infected by consuming contaminated meat that is not fully cooked or by directly ingesting infectious particles. Cat feces may contain large quantities of infectious particles, making these animals an important source of infection. In rare instances, toxoplasmosis is acquired through blood transfusion.

In most people, toxoplasmosis occurs asymptomatically or causes mild disease. In persons with normal immune responses, *Toxoplasma* infection occasionally causes an infectious mononucleosislike illness with fever, swelling of lymph glands, and rash. In persons with impaired immune responses, however, such as persons with AIDS, toxoplasmosis can be a serious, life-threatening illness.

If a nonimmune pregnant woman ingests infectious *T gondii* particles, they enter her blood stream and are carried to the placenta. Approximately one third of fetuses of infected mothers are themselves infected with these organisms. Whether the fetus becomes infected depends primarily on the stage of pregnancy at which maternal infection takes place. Most serious fetal infections are the result of toxoplasmosis infection during the second trimester of pregnancy.

Approximately 5% of fetal infections with *T gondii* result in stillbirth or miscarriage. Most infants who survive fetal toxoplasmosis infection have no symptoms at birth, although some infected infants later show abnormalities of the eyes (chorioretinitis) or hydrocephalus. Approximately 25% to 30% of infected newborns have symptoms in infancy. The spectrum of abnormalities caused by *T gondii* (see Table 14-1) resembles that of congenital CMV infection. Both agents damage the brain and eyes.

A diagnosis of toxoplasmosis can usually be established by performing blood tests on the infant and mother. These tests measure antibodies to the toxoplasma organisms. If the level of antibody is high or shows a fourfold or greater increase soon after birth, toxoplasmosis is likely. These antibody tests detect only about 75% of actual toxoplasma infections. A diagnosis of *Toxoplasmosis* can be confirmed by identifying *Toxoplasma* organisms within human cells during autopsy or analysis of pathologic tissues.

Many different medical strategies have been developed to combat congenital toxoplasmosis. In certain regions of the world, the diagnosis can be established before the infant's birth, and the mother can be treated with anti-toxoplasma medications. This approach seems to diminish the potential for fetal damage. It is currently recommended that live-born infected infants with signs of congenital toxoplasmosis be treated with a combination of antibiotics that kills the *Toxoplasma* organisms and may therefore preclude further damage to tissues.

The risk of congenital toxoplasmosis might be reduced by avoiding cats or poorly cooked meat. Because toxoplasmosis is not acquired from person-to-person contact, infants with congenital toxoplasmosis pose no risk to exposed children or adults.

OTHER AGENTS

Enteroviruses

Before polio vaccines were developed, poliovirus (an enterovirus that causes infantile paralysis) infection during pregnancy occasionally caused stillbirth, miscarriage, or congenital malformation. Other enteroviral infections, although common among pregnant women, rarely result in congenital infection and birth defects. Enteroviral infections that the infant acquires (often from the mother) around the time of birth, however, can produce illnesses ranging from mild to fatal. Some perinatal enterovirus infections cause signs and symptoms similar to those caused by disseminated HSV infection, and mortality among severe cases ranges from 10% to 20%.

Enteroviruses are highly contagious agents that often cause communitywide epidemics. Such infections, although common, pose little risk to most healthy children and adults. Women in their last trimester of pregnancy, however, should avoid contact with children who have proven or suspected enteroviral infections.

Varicella-Zoster (Chickenpox, Shingles) Virus

The varicella-zoster virus, another member of the herpesvirus family, can also cause congenital infection. Because chickenpox infections usually take place during childhood and seldom during pregnancy, however, this type of congenital infection is uncommon.

Congenital varicella infection of the fetus, like other congenital viral infections, occurs during maternal infection and results from passage of the virus across the placenta. The infection may cause miscarriage, stillbirth, or damage to various fetal tissues. Abnormalities attributed to congenital varicella include scarring of the skin, shortened or paralyzed limbs, cataracts, microcephaly, and low birth weight.

If maternal chickenpox occurs within 4 or 5 days of delivery, the newborn infant can have widespread infection involving the liver, lungs, brain, and kidneys. As many as 30% of newborns with varicella infection died before the era of antiviral therapy. Some infants exposed to persons with chickenpox may require intervention with varicella-zoster immune globulin, a serum that contains antibodies to this virus. If infants (or children) become infected with the varicella-zoster virus, therapy with an antiviral drug (acyclovir) can be beneficial. Acyclovir is not generally recommended for all children, however. Providers should contact a pediatrician for the latest recommendations.

Infants with varicella-zoster infections can transmit the disease when they have active skin vesicles. These infants, like older children with chickenpox, should be isolated from other infants or nonimmune children and adults until the skin lesions are crusted over.

Human Parvovirus B19

Human parvovirus B19, the causative agent of fifth disease (a childhood illness associated with fever and slapped-cheek rash) can occasionally infect a nonimmune pregnant woman and damage the fetus. Human parvovirus B19 can cause stillbirth or severe anemia resulting in extreme swelling (edema) of fetal tissues, or it may produce no adverse effects on the fetus. Most pregnant women who become infected with human parvovirus B19 give birth to normal infants.

Lyme Disease

Infection with *Borrelia burgdorferi*, the cause of Lyme disease, during pregnancy has been associated with fetal infection leading to death or congenital heart disease. Congenital infection with *burgdorferi* appears to be uncommon.

RUBELLA

Until the late 1960s, rubella (also called German measles or 3-day measles) was the most common viral cause of birth defects in children. During epidemics, as many as 1 in every 200 live-born infants had organ damage as a result of maternal infection with the rubella virus. After licensure of the live attenuated rubella vaccine in 1969, however, the incidence of congenital rubella syndrome dropped to fewer than 1 case per 10,000 live births. Congenital rubella syndrome reappeared in the United States during the 1980s as a result of a lack of universal immunity among women of childbearing age.

In both children and adults, rubella produces only a mild systemic illness with fever, rash, and respiratory symptoms. If a woman is infected during her first trimester of pregnancy, however, there is a high likelihood of damage to developing fetal organs. By contrast, the infant infrequently has signs of rubella infection when maternal infection occurs after the fourth month.

Like other congenital infections, rubella can cause miscarriage or stillbirth. More often, however, the infant survives and has damage to many tissues, including the eyes, brain, heart, liver, lungs, kidneys, skin, bones, and hormone-secreting organs. The tissues most commonly affected are the eyes, brain, and heart. The infant may have cataracts, small eyes (microphthalmia), inflammation of the retina (chorioretinitis), encephalitis, microcephaly, and congenital heart defects (usually patent ductus arteriosus). Rubella-infected infants often have a skin rash, a feature that reflects a reduced platelet count and bleeding into the skin.

Nearly all infected infants with signs or symptoms of rubella will have some degree of long-term neurologic impairment. Like CMV, rubella can damage the inner ear and produce nerve deafness. Many asymptomatic infants born to mothers who had rubella infection during pregnancy later develop deafness or psychomotor retardation. In addition, rubella-infected infants occasionally manifest thyroid dysfunction, growth disturbance, or diabetes mellitus.

Although no effective antiviral therapy is available to treat congenital rubella infection in newborns, rubella can be prevented by vaccination. The rubella vaccine should be included in all childhood immunization programs. In addition, women of childbearing age should have their blood tested to ascertain whether they are immune to rubella. If they are not, they should receive the rubella vaccine at a time when they are not pregnant.

Children with congenital rubella should be excluded from center-based programs until throat and urine cultures are negative for the rubella virus. Pregnant women who have not had rubella or have not received rubella immunization should avoid contact with infants with congenital rubella. Excretion of the virus diminishes greatly during the first year of life. Thereafter, these children pose little or no risk to nonimmune pregnant women.

CYTOMEGALOVIRUS

CMV infection occurs before birth in approximately 1 of every 100 liveborn infants, making CMV the most common congenital infection worldwide. Only 10% to 20% of infected infants have signs or symptoms attributable to CMV, and only half of these have a serious disorder that has been known historically as cytomegalic inclusion disease.

Human CMV infection occurs throughout the world in people of all ages. In the United States, most adults possess antibodies to CMV, indicating prior exposure to the virus. Approximately 30% to 60% of women of childbearing age in the United States lack immunity to CMV, however. By contrast, people in developing nations or highly populated areas tend to acquire CMV in childhood, presumably through direct contact with CMV-excreting playmates.

The manifestations of CMV infection depend on the age and immune status of the infected individual. In healthy children and adults, including pregnant women, CMV infection rarely causes symptoms, although occasionally an infectious mononucleosis-like illness develops with fever, fatigue, and swelling of the lymph nodes. By contrast, people with impaired immune systems (eg, organ transplant recipients or persons with AIDS) can develop serious complications, such as pneumonia, eye infection, or encephalitis.

The majority of congenitally infected infants have no symptoms at birth (the infection is recognizable by the excretion of CMV in the urine). Even so, 10% to 15% of these infected but asymptomatic infants later develop hearing loss caused by chronic CMV infection of the inner ear, and some children may also have subtle behavioral or developmental consequences.

Approximately 5% to 10% of congenitally infected infants have a serious and sometimes fatal condition characterized by damage to numerous body organs, including the brain, lungs, and liver (see Table 14-1). CMV also causes jaundice, skin rash, abnormal blood and platelet counts, enlargement of the spleen, and eye damage (chorioretinitis).

By far the most serious consequence of symptomatic CMV infection is damage to the developing brain. The most common abnormality in infants with severe CMV infection is deficient brain growth manifested by a small head size (microcephaly). Survivors of symptomatic CMV infection often have substantial neurologic impairments, including developmental and mental retardation, motor abnormalities, seizures, visual deficits, and nerve deafness.

Currently, CMV infection can be neither prevented nor effectively treated. None of the available antiviral agents has proved to be effective against congenital CMV infection, although newer antiviral drugs are currently being investigated. There is no vaccine that can prevent birth defects due to congenital CMV infection.

CMV is present in the urine, saliva, blood, cervical secretions, and semen of infected individuals. The urine and saliva usually contain the largest quantities of viral particles, and the virus can be shed for months or even years. Transmission of CMV results from close, personal contact with infected individuals, often children or sexual partners. Mothers can transmit CMV to their nursing children via breast milk, and transfused persons can acquire CMV from infected blood products.

In the United States and other western countries, 10% to 20% of otherwise healthy l-year-olds excrete CMV. In some day care centers, as many as 70% of children between the ages of 1 and 3 years excrete CMV. The risk of acquiring CMV varies according to the nature of the contact with CMV-infected children. Persons who work with children in hospitals have low rates of infection, whereas day care workers or parents of CMV-excreting young children have relatively high rates of CMV infection (see Chapters 5 and 6).

Pregnant women should avoid daily, hands-on contact with infants or young children with known congenital CMV infection. The risk may be greatest during the child's first year of life, when large quantities of the virus are excreted in urine or saliva. Approximately 50% of children with congenital CMV infection continue to shed virus in their urine for 4 years or more.

Any young child, especially one attending group day care, may be excreting CMV. Consequently, women who have contact with young children and anticipate pregnancy in the future should know their CMV immune status. This can be determined by a blood test (CMV serology), which a physician can order. Pregnant women who are seronegative and therefore not immune to CMV should limit their exposure to toddler-age children (who are more likely to be excreting CMV) and should practice good hygiene, by washing their hands after contact with children or their secretions, and by avoiding oral contact (eg, kissing or food sharing) with the children or their secretions (see Chapter 6).

HERPES SIMPLEX VIRUS

HSV causes serious illness in 1 in every 10,000 live-born infants. This virus exists in two forms: HSV type 1, which causes cold sores and gingivostomatitis, and HSV type 2, which causes most genital herpetic lesions. Most cases of perinatal HSV infections are caused by HSV type 2.

Unlike CMV and *Toxoplasma gaondii,* which are acquired prior to birth, HSV infections are usually acquired perinatally; that is, they occur during or shortly after birth. Although HSV can be transmitted to the fetus via the placenta or amniotic fluid, most infections occur when the infant passes through the birth canal of a mother who has been infected with HSV and has HSV in her cervical or vaginal secretions. Less often, the infant contracts HSV from an adult who has active oral herpes.

Symptoms of perinatal HSV infection usually begin during the first 5 to 7 days of life and vary according to the distribution of the disease. In approximately 40% of cases, infection is localized to the skin, mouth, or eye, causing blisters (vesicles) of the skin or mouth (see Color Plate 10) or inflammation of the cornea. In another 35%, infection is restricted to the brain (herpes encephalitis) with lethargy or irritability and serious neurologic signs, such as seizures or coma. In as many as 25% of cases, the infection is disseminated throughout the infant's body, causing fever, vomiting, jaundice, lethargy, skin vesicles, and involvement of the liver or spleen (see Table 14-1).

The development of acyclovir and vidarabine, two effective anti-HSV drugs, has reduced overall mortality in neonatal HSV infections to 40% or less. The prognosis for an HSV-infected infant depends on the extent of the disease and the prompt initiation of anti-HSV therapy. For example, infants with localized infection of the skin do well with little mortality or long-term effects. By contrast, half the infants with severe, disseminated HSV infections die, and 20% to 30% of the survivors have long-term impairments ranging from poor growth to seizures, blindness, and mental retardation.

Some instances of perinatal HSV infection can be prevented. If active genital herpes lesions are present at the time of the mother's labor, the infant should be delivered by cesarean section, particularly if the bag of waters (amniotic membrane) has not ruptured (less than half the mothers who give birth to infants with HSV have either a history of genital HSV infection or evidence of this condition, such as genital lesions). All infants younger than 2 months should be isolated from adults who have active oral herpes lesions. Any adult with active oral herpes should wear a protective mask when caring for infants younger than 1 month.

Infants with HSV infections who have active, noncrusted vesicles on exposed skin should be excluded from center-based programs. Exclusion is not necessary if the infected area can be covered by clothing or protective bandages. Children with oral herpes lesions can participate in center-based programs if they can control their oral secretions.

Personnel who work with HSV-infected infants at home should wear gloves when the infants have fresh (active) skin vesicles because these contain considerable amounts of infectious virus. When the lesions are crusted or absent, these infants pose no risk to exposed personnel and can attend school or day care centers.

GENERAL RECOMMENDATIONS FOR ALL CONGENITAL INFECTIONS

Children who survive congenital infections often have multiple long-term complications that require a multidisciplinary approach to treatment guided by a developmental pediatrician or pediatric neurologist. Many medical services may be required, including those of an eye specialist (ophthalmologist), bone and joint surgeon (orthopedist), and hearing specialist (audiologist).

Children with developmental delay require early intervention programs. Intelligence testing with age-appropriate instruments should be performed as early as reliable results can be obtained. Because visual abnormalities are common complications of congenital infections, affected children should be examined by a pediatric ophthalmologist.

Because many congenital infections are associated with nerve deafness (sensorineural deafness), periodic audiologic testing is important. Some children, particularly those infected with CMV or rubella virus, can develop progressive or new-onset hearing loss. A conservative approach is to perform audiometric testing at birth, at 6 months, at 1 year, and annually thereafter until the child reaches school age. Many children will benefit from hearing aids. Deafness is sometimes so severe, however, that the child requires special supportive services throughout the school years and beyond.

As with nearly all infections, the risk of transmitting infection from certain congenitally infected infants can be greatly diminished by good hygiene. Diapers should be promptly discarded in appropriate containers. Also, personnel should wash their hands well after contact with infected infants. Gloves need not be worn except when one is handling infants with active HSV or varicella zoster skin lesions or changing the diapers of infants with CMV infection.

REFERENCES

Baldwin S, Whitley RJ. Teratogen update: intrauterine herpes simplex virus infection. *Teratology*. 1989; 39:1–10

Bale JF Jr, Murph JR. Congenital infections and the nervous system. *Pediatr Clin North Am*. 1992; 39:669–690.

Blackman JA, Andersen RD, Healy A, Zehrbach R. Management of young children with recurrent herpes simplex skin lesions in special education programs. *Pediatr Infect Dis J*. 1985; 4:221–224.

DesMonts G, Couvreur J. Congenital toxoplasmosis: a prospective study of 378 pregnancies. *N Engl J Med*. 1974; 290:1110–1116.

Hanshaw JB, Dudgeon JA. *Viral Diseases of the Fetus and Newborn*. Philadelphia, Pa: Saunders; 1985.

Nahmias AJ. The TORCH complex. *Hospital Pract*. 1974; pp.65–72.

Rolfs RT, Nakashima AK. Epidemiology of primary and secondary syphilis in the United States, 1981 through 1989. *JAMA*. 1990; 264:1432–1437.

Zenker PN, Berman SM. Congenital syphilis: trends and recommendations for evaluation and management. *Pediatr Infect Dis J*. 1991; 10:516–522.

Chapter 15

Acquired Immunodeficiency Syndrome

Acquired immunodeficiency syndrome (AIDS) was first observed in the United States in the early 1980s. In the ensuing decade, this disease grew to massive national and international proportions. It is believed that the causative viral agent currently infects more than one million Americans and tens of millions worldwide.

AIDS is the term for the later stage of infection with human immunodeficiency virus (HIV), in which the immune system is seriously impaired. There is increasing susceptibility to infectious and malignant diseases ultimately resulting in death. Although there is no known cure, antiviral treatment strategies are expanding and prolonging life. There is wide variation among individuals in the speed of progression of disease.

After the first cases of AIDS were described in 1981, the disease was observed almost exclusively in homosexual and bisexual men, intravenous drug users, prostitutes, hemophiliacs, and others receiving blood products. Since 1985, screening of blood has dramatically reduced blood-related HIV acquisition, but the virus has infected increasing numbers of heterosexual persons and children of HIV-infected mothers.

CAUSE

The cause of AIDS and related conditions is HIV, which is now recognized as having more than one type. The virus (formerly termed HTLV-III or LAV) brings about insidious alterations in immune regulation and function by infecting a type of white blood cell known as helper or CD4 lymphocytes. Other cells of the body may be infected to various degrees, and the virus has been cultured from most body fluids, including blood, semen, saliva, and tears.

An infected individual may not develop symptoms for months or years after the initial infection, yet the virus is harbored in the body and can potentially infect others. The principal modes of transmission are intimate sexual contact (multiple sexual partners increase the risk) and shared contaminated needles. Infected mothers can transmit the agent to their offspring during pregnancy or during the birth process. Therefore, the offspring of women who have antibodies to HIV are at risk for developing the disease. Because of the decline of blood product–acquired HIV infection, mother–infant transmission has become virtually the only route of HIV acquisition for young children in the United States.

SIGNS AND SYMPTOMS

HIV produces a spectrum of illness ranging from few or no symptoms to the later, severe manifestation called AIDS. How severely a person is affected may depend on personal and environmental factors.

Many of the signs and symptoms of AIDS result, directly or indirectly, from injury to the immune system. In the adult, these may include profound fatigue, persistent fevers, diminished appetite, weight loss, enlarged lymph nodes, dry cough, persistent diarrhea, thrush (a whitish yeast infection of the mouth), a tendency to bruise easily, and purplish or discolored growths on or beneath the skin or mucous membranes of the mouth, anus, nasal passages, or under the eyelids.

The symptoms are somewhat more variable and nonspecific in children. The most common features are failure to thrive, developmental delay, enlarged liver and spleen, chronic diarrhea, upper respiratory infections, ear infections, thrush, and recurrent pneumonias. Children with AIDS are also prone to serious, life-threatening bacterial infections such as meningitis, pneumonia, and infection of the blood (sepsis).

The first sign of AIDS in the adult is often a fever that may last weeks or months and is followed by the onset of rather unusual infections or malignancies. One such infection is a pneumonia caused by *Pneumocystis carinii*, a protozoan that usually affects only persons whose defense mechanisms are compromised by severe malnutrition or chemotherapy for cancer. A malignancy often seen in adults with AIDS is an otherwise rare cancer called Kaposi's sarcoma, manifested by the discolored growths described above.

DIAGNOSIS

AIDS is diagnosed primarily on the clinical signs and symptoms of the disease, but laboratory test results may clarify the immune status. The first test for persons who manifest symptoms of AIDS, and for those who have been exposed to the virus or who belong to a high-risk group, is for specific antibodies in the blood. In response to infectious organisms, certain blood cells called lymphocytes produce antibodies that attach to the invaders, enabling other cells to capture and destroy them. When exposed to HIV, lymphocytes produce antibodies specifically directed toward this virus. These antibodies can be detected by a simple, inexpensive blood test. This is not a test for AIDS but for antibodies to the virus that causes AIDS.

Tests for antibodies to HIV are generally accurate. Even so, they may yield positive results when there are no antibodies present; conversely, the results may rarely be negative despite the presence of HIV infection. Other, more specific tests for AIDS involve culturing HIV itself from body fluids such as blood, saliva, and semen and measuring viral products. Tests of the various components of the immune system can also aid in diagnosis. The physician can look for abnormalities of the immune system that are more typical of AIDS than of other immunologic disorders.

Diagnosis of HIV infection in infants born to HIV-infected mothers may take weeks or months. Roughly two thirds of all such infants escape HIV acquisition altogether. Because maternal antibodies to HIV (and other infectious agents) may be present for up to 15 months in the infant, tests other than antibody tests are utilized to confirm or rule out infection.

MANAGEMENT

The critical question for caretakers and parents is whether an HIV-infected child poses a risk to others in a foster home, day care setting, early invention program, or school. Experience to date provides great reassurance regarding the improbability of such transmission.

First, HIV is clearly less communicable than hepatitis B, cytomegalovirus, and other agents known to be transmitted in group child care. Second, the virtual absence of sibling-to-sibling transmission, even with such intimate involvement as toothbrush sharing, implies no measurable risk through usual day care contact. Third, although virus is found in saliva, the contagious potential of saliva appears to be negligible, especially in comparison to that of blood or semen. Finally, experience in the health care setting implies that exposure to blood (eg, via needle stick) is a virtual prerequisite for transmission.

Usual hygienic measures and the adoption of universal precautions for all blood spills in the school or child care setting should suffice in maintaining the theoretical risk of HIV transmission at or near zero. A decade of experience without HIV transmission in child care environments should reassure parents and caretakers dealing with known HIV-infected children.

A more appropriate focus may be the risk of other children's infections to the HIV-infected infant or child. Medical management of HIV-infected children involves an increasing number of preventive measures, including antibiotic prophylaxis and immune globulin infusions. Although some infection risk is independent of contact with others, it is prudent and reasonable to reduce the contact of children with AIDS with other children known to be ill with routine childhood illnesses.

Some medical interventions, such as antiviral medication, may be at sufficiently frequent intervals to necessitate medication during the school day. Providers may need to familiarize themselves with these medications and their side effects. The number and complexity of medications are likely to increase in coming years.

Beyond infection risk, the other realm of greatest importance to providers caring for HIV-infected children is that pertaining to neurologic development. Because HIV infection may result in various neurologic and behavioral alterations, providers will need to work closely with parents and health care personnel in assessing the child's status and needs.

It is important to encourage adequate caloric and nutrient intake because poor nutrition can further compromise the immune system or adversely affect neurologic development. Sometimes children with AIDS must receive their nutrition directly through the veins (intravenous alimentation). This procedure can provide a direct route for other infectious organisms to enter the body. Management for AIDS may include dietary supplements to ensure intake of the large amounts of calories and nutrients necessary for a child with chronic illness.

COMPLICATIONS

In both children and adults with AIDS, the complications result from the body's inability to mount an appropriate immune response to foreign substances. All age groups are susceptible to unusual infections, such as the pneumonia caused by the protozoan *Pneumocystis carinii* and oral yeast infections (thrush or candidiasis). Because infants have not had a chance to develop antibodies to common bacteria, they are prone to serious bacterial infections as well. Infants have also been reported to contract cancer, although malignancies are more common among adults. The final consequence of AIDS appears to be death due to infection or cancer. In the meantime, children experience poor growth, recurrent infections, diarrhea, and the social stigma that accompanies the disease.

RECOMMENDATIONS

Children with AIDS should be provided with as normal an environment as possible, including opportunities for social, emotional, and developmental nurturing. School or day care settings may, however, increase the affected child's exposure to infectious agents against which the impaired immune system is not effective. Because children with AIDS are more susceptible to infections, they should be kept away from others with illnesses. Signs of illness (eg, fever, irritability, or changes in behavior) should be reported to a nurse or physician promptly.

For most infected school-age children, the benefits of an unrestricted setting outweigh the risks of acquiring potentially harmful infections. Moreover, there is apparently no risk of these children transmitting HIV. Therefore, they should generally be allowed to attend school and after-school activities. Universal precautions with respect to blood spills should permit safe involvement in athletic activities.

The group care setting for infants and preschoolers has been scrutinized for HIV infection because of the frequency of transmission of other agents. The lack of documented transmission provides a basis for a continued posture favoring attendance by HIV-infected infants and toddlers. Usual hygienic measures, universal blood precautions, and special considerations for children who bite remain appropriate.

Good hygienic practices are prudent in caring for children with AIDS. Care providers should wash their hands with soap after intimate contact, dispose of diapers and waste products properly, and disinfect toys and other objects that may have virus-containing saliva on them (use 1 part chlorine bleach to 10 parts water). As an additional barrier to possible but unlikely transmission, disposable gloves could be worn when one is handling infected children, especially if exposure to blood or body fluids is likely. Although holding and cuddling infants and young children with AIDS appear to be safe practices, kissing in such a way that the child's saliva comes into contact with the caretaker's mouth poses unnecessary risk.

Good nutrition is important. A dietitian can help develop a plan for a child who may have a poor appetite yet who needs more than the usual number of calories because of chronic illness. Supplements to the diet can provide a high number of calories and nutrients in relatively small quantities of food.

Because the child with AIDS may be from a deprived social situation, social workers and other support personnel should assist parents and caretakers with the complex and expensive medical management problems caused by this disease. Providers should be aware of and seek involvement of appropriate local resources for HIV-infected children and their families.

REFERENCES

Baker LS. *You and H.I.V. A Day at a Time.* Philadelphia, PA: Saunders; 1991.

Education and foster care of children infected with Human T-Lymphotropic Virus Type III/ Lymphadenopathy-Associated Virus. *MMWR.* 1985; 34:517–521.

Schinazi RF, Nahmias AJ. *AIDS in Children, Adolescents, and Heterosexual Adults.* New York, NY: Elsevier Science Publishing Co.; 1988.

Chapter 16

Parasites

Parasites live on or in the body, deriving sustenance from the host. They frequently attach themselves to a particular body part, which they prefer over other body parts or tissue types. Most parasitic infestations are not life threatening, but they can cause irritating symptoms, such as diarrhea and itching. Some parasites are transmitted through direct person-to-person contact; others are transmitted through contaminated food and water. A few are carried by pets. Because of the potential for spread among children and child care providers, control of parasites in day care and educational settings demands a systematic—and calm—approach.

PARASITES OF THE SKIN (DERMATOPHYTES)

Fungi

Ringworm of the Scalp

Ringworm of the scalp (tinea capitis) is infection by a fungus, not a worm, that can be acquired from contact with infected persons, animals (including household pets), or soil. The affected areas of the scalp are well-demarcated, scaly patches where hair has broken off or fallen out (see Color Plate 11). This disease should always be considered in children with areas of baldness (alopecia).

Often there is no discomfort with ringworm, but some individuals develop an allergic response to the fungus with resulting inflammation, itching, and secondary bacterial infection.

Diagnosis can sometimes be made by shining a special light over the affected areas because some species of the fungus give off a typical fluorescence. Other species can be seen under the microscope and cultured in the laboratory. Ringworm of the scalp is treated with antifungal medication (eg, griseofulvin), which is taken orally for 4 to 8 weeks. In addition, a topical ointment may be applied. Although the fungus is not readily transmitted, close contact with other children is not advisable until treatment is successfully completed.

Ringworm of the Body

Ringworm of the body (tinea corporis) is an infection of the skin by a fungus, not by a worm. It appears as circular, red, scaly patches that spread along the outer circumference, leaving the inner area of the circle clear. The fungus can usually be identified by microscopic examination of the scales. Applying a topical antifungal ointment (eg, Monistat®, Lotrimin®, and Mycelex®) for 2 to 4 weeks is usually sufficient to eradicate the infection. In extreme cases, oral medication may be necessary.

Athlete's Foot

Fungal infections of the foot (tinea pedis, or athlete's foot) are characterized by a softening, thinning, and cracking of the skin, especially around and between the toes. This annoying condition, which is relatively uncommon in preadolescent children, is treated with a topical antifungal ointment (eg, Tinactin®, Micatin®, or Monistat®).

Thrush and Monilial Diaper Rash

A yeastlike fungus (*Candida albicans*) commonly causes infection in the diaper area, which is called monilial diaper rash (moniliasis), and in the mouth, which is called thrush (candidiasis).

Monilial diaper rash is a bright red, well-demarcated, moist, nontender rash that occurs in the genital area and around the buttocks, extending down onto the thighs. Beyond the outer edges of this confluent rash are often small, scattered, pus-filled lesions. Monilial diaper rash can be confused with, or occur simultaneously with, other rashes. Therefore, proper diagnosis and treatment (a topical nystatin-containing ointment) require an experienced practitioner. No special precautions are necessary to prevent spread of this fungus.

Thrush is discussed in Chapter 7.

Arthropods

Lice

Head lice (which cause pediculosis capitis) are small, wingless parasites that infest the hair of the scalp and occasionally the eyebrows and lashes. They feed on blood and die within 2 or 3 days after they are removed from the body. The lice themselves may not be readily visible, but the eggs can be seen sticking to the hairs, where they reach maturity within 2 or 3 weeks (see Color Plate 12).

Itching is the most common symptom of head lice, although children with mild infestations may not complain. Secretions from the bites can trigger inflammation and produce a raised rash on the scalp. If this rash is scratched, it can become infected with bacteria, causing pus-filled or weepy lesions.

Infestations are treated with lice-killing shampoos, which may need to be applied repeatedly (eg, Kwell® or RID®) or once (eg, Nix®) to kill the eggs and lice. Eggs that stick to hair shafts after treatment are usually not alive. Because of concerns about reinfestation or inadequate treatment, however, most schools and day care centers enforce a "no-nit" return policy. Therefore, eggs can be removed with a fine-toothed comb to permit later examination for reinfestation or inadequate treatment. To prevent reinfestation, clothing and used bedding should be washed in hot water and/or dried on the hot cycle. Dry cleaning or storage in plastic bags for 10 days is also effective.

Head lice epidemics occur worldwide and among all socioeconomic groups. Infestation is not an indication of uncleanliness. Transmission occurs by direct contact with infested individuals or indirectly through contact with personal articles, such as clothing or hair brushes, that may contain lice. Isolation of infested individuals is not necessary after the first treatment is given.

During epidemics, contacts in the home and in the school or day care setting should be examined for signs of infestation. A calm approach to managing head lice can do much to prevent unwarranted panic, recriminations, and calls from irate parents.

Ticks

Most tick bites cause no problems beyond skin irritation. Occasionally, however, a tick bite can lead to serious diseases, such as Rocky Mountain spotted fever, Lyme disease (see Chapter 17), or tick paralysis. Worldwide, ticks are second only to mosquitos as arthropod transmitters of human disease.

Ehrlichiosis. An increasingly recognized disease transmitted to humans through tick bites is ehrlichiosis, caused by the rickettsial organism *ehrlichia canis*. The symptoms are similar to those of Rocky Mountain Spotted fever—fever, chills, headache, muscle and joint pain, nausea, and vomiting. A rash usually occurs about a week after onset of the illness. The illness can last up to two weeks and recovery is usually complete. Most cases have occurred from May through July in the southeastern and southcentral regions of the U.S., but the disease seems to be spreading. Tetracycline for children nine or older and chloramphenicol are effective methods of treatment. No special isolation procedures are needed.

The following are recommendations from the American Academy of Pediatrics for prevention of tick-borne infections.

- Avoid tick-infested areas whenever possible.
- Protective clothing that covers the arms, legs, and other exposed areas should be worn if a tick-infested area is entered. Other protective measures include tucking pants into boots or socks and buttoning long-sleeved shirts at the cuff. Permethrin (RID® spray) may be sprayed onto clothes and is effective in decreasing tick attachment.
- Tick and insect repellents such as deet applied to the skin provide additional protection but require reapplication every 1 to 2 hours for effectiveness. If deet is used it should be applied sparingly and only to exposed skin. Seizures in young children have been reported coincident with its application. It should not be applied to irritated or abraded skin or on a child's hands, and it should be washed off after the child comes indoors.
- Persons should be taught to inspect themselves and their clothing daily after possible tick exposure. Special attention should be given to the exposed hairy regions of the body where ticks like to attach.
- Ticks should be removed promptly. Care should be taken to avoid squeezing the body of the tick because transmission of infection can result. The tick should be grasped with a fine tweezer close to the skin and removed by carefully pulling. If the fingers are used to remove ticks, they should be protected with facial tissue and washed afterward.
- A tick that is not removed within a few hours is a potential source of serious disease. Prompt, careful removal can usually prevent problems.
- Daily inspection of pets and removal of any ticks is advised.

In tick-borne illnesses, symptoms may not appear for a week or 10 days. If a child who has been bitten by a tick shows any signs of illness during that period, a physician should be notified.

Mosquitos

When taking their blood meal, female mosquitos—like ticks, lice, horseflies, and fleas—introduce saliva into the skin. This can produce an allergic response, resulting in localized itching. Mosquitos can also carry organisms that cause encephalitis (see Chapter 9), malaria, yellow fever, or other diseases.

Scabies

Scabies is an intensely itchy skin rash caused by a mite (*Sarcoptes scabiei*), a small insect in the spider family. In older children and adults a rash of raised red bumps occurs, usually between the fingers but often on the wrists, elbows, belt line, thighs, and genitals. In infants, the rash is more likely to occur on the head, neck, palms, and soles (see Color Plate 13). If it has not been obliterated by scratching, the mite's burrow appears as a short, wavy, dirty line at the center of each cluster of red bumps.

Itching is often most intense at night. Children who have not had scabies before may not experience itching for 2 to 6 weeks after exposure to mites. Those with previous exposure develop this symptom far more quickly, usually within several days. Diagnosis is based on the appearance of the rash and complaints of itching (or visible scratch marks). Scrapings of affected areas reveal the mite under the microscope.

Scabies occurs worldwide and can affect all socioeconomic classes, although it is more common where there is poverty, poor sanitation, and crowding. Transmission can occur as long as the infected person goes untreated.

Several medications that are effective against mites are lindane (Kwell® and Scabene®), permethrin (Elimite®) and crotomiton (Eurax®). Their use, especially in infants, should be supervised by a physician.

Chiggers

The larva of the harvest mite, which is common in the southern and midwestern states, is a tiny red parasite that creeps into skin pores and hair follicles to feed, causing a rash and immediate itching. Insect repellents offer protection against chiggers, and topical steroids help relieve itching.

PARASITES OF THE GASTROINTESTINAL TRACT

Giardiasis

Giardia lamblia, which is prevalent worldwide, is a protozoan that can cause foul-smelling diarrhea and gas, bloating, appetite loss, and growth failure. In some cases, there may be no symptoms at all. In fact, studies have shown that in day care centers as many as 20% of children younger than 3 years carry this organism without having symptoms.

The cysts of the organism are transmitted through fecal contamination of food and water. Most epidemics result from contaminated water supplies, such as shallow wells into which surface water drains. Person-to-person transmission can occur, especially in day care or institutional settings serving children who are not toilet trained. Individuals are infectious as long as they are excreting cysts of the organism in their feces.

This parasite is detectable by microscopic examination of stool specimens. It is sometimes necessary to examine many stool specimens or to obtain fluid from the upper part of the intestine, where the organism resides. Take-home kits with chemicals in child-proof containers are available for the convenient collection of multiple stool specimens. Oral drugs (eg, Furoxone®, Flagyl®, and Atabrine®) can eradicate the organism. Treated children can return to the school or day care center after the diarrhea has ceased.

Hand washing by staff and children is important, especially after toilet use or diaper changes. It does not take many organisms to cause a new infection. During epidemics, consultation with public health authorities may be necessary to help prevent spreading and to determine, if possible, the source(s) of infection.

Amebiasis

Amebiasis is caused by the protozoan *Entamoeba histolytica*. Most infections produce no symptoms or only mild intestinal problems, such as bloating, constipation, or loose stools. Sometimes, however, an affected child has acute diarrhea with abdominal cramping. In severe cases, there may be bloody, mucous stools, abdominal pain, fever, headache, and chills. Infection occurs through contact with feces that contain the cysts of the organism (sometimes these are found in contaminated water).

Diagnosis is made by examining the stool under the microscope. Various oral drugs are used for treatment. No isolation procedures are necessary, but good hand washing and proper disposal of human waste are important. In investigating the source of the infection, all individuals who come into close contact with the child should be screened because asymptomatic individuals may be spreading the organism unknowingly.

Cryptosporidiosis

Outbreaks of diarrhea in day care centers can be caused by the protozoan *Cryptosporidium*. Usually, the diarrhea lasts about 10 days. Children with poor immunity can develop chronic, severe diarrhea with malnutrition and dehydration, however. The diagnosis can be made by microscopic examination of the stool for the organism. There is usually not specific treatment other than fluid replacement. Precautions should be taken to prevent person-to-person transmission of this parasite through hand washing and proper disposal of diapers. The parasite is not affected by chlorine and is not always removed by water filters.

Pinworms

Pinworms (*Enterobius vermicularis,* also called threadworms or seatworms) infest children throughout the world and in all socioeconomic groups. Up to 15% of the US population is infested at any one time. An especially high rate of infestation is found among young children and their families and among institutionalized children.

When eggs are swallowed, they pass down the digestive tract and hatch in the upper intestine. The escaping larvae migrate to the lower intestine, where they attach to the wall and mature to adulthood within 3 or 4 weeks. Pregnant worms crawl out the anus, usually at night, to lay eggs. This activity causes intense itching, and the child scratches the anal area, gets eggs on the fingertips, and later puts the fingers in the mouth, starting the cycle all over again. Eggs may also be introduced into the mouth through contact with contaminated objects, such as clothing. In girls, the worms may infect the vagina, causing irritation and inflammation (see Chapter 11).

Pinworm infection (enterobiasis) is diagnosed by applying transparent adhesive tape to the anal area to pick up any eggs and then applying this tape to a glass slide for examination under a microscope. If the child's anal area is examined during the night, the worms themselves can be seen coming out to lay their eggs.

Pinworms can be effectively eradicated by drugs (eg, Antiminth®, Vermox®, Antepar®, or Povan®). Because spread within the family is common, some physicians prefer to treat the entire family of a child with pinworms.

Table 16-1 Other Parasitic Worms

Name	*Organism*	*Route of entry*	*Means of transmission*	*Symptoms*	*Treatment*	*Precautions*
Hookworm	*Necator americanus*	Larvae enter through skin, especially feet, after contact with infected soil. Larvae migrate in the blood to lungs, are coughed up and swallowed, and attach to intestinal wall, laying new eggs	Infected soil	None to mild	Drugs	Sanitary disposal of feces, wearing shoes in endemic areas
Strongyloidiasis	*Strongyloides stercoralis*	Same as hookworm	Infected soil	Cough, abdominal pain, vomiting, diarrhea	Drugs	Same as hookworm
Whipworm	*Trichuris trichiura*	Eggs are ingested and swallowed, hatch in upper intestine, reach adulthood, and lay eggs	Infected soil	Often none; failure to thrive, diarrhea	Drugs	Sanitary disposal of feces, good hand washing before meals
Visceral larva migrans	*Toxocara canis* (dog roundworm) *Toxocara cati* (cat roundworm)	Eggs are ingested and swallowed and hatch in upper intestine. Larvae migrate through intestinal wall and reach various organs (lungs, liver, eyes, brain), where they fail to mature, die, and cause inflammation	Soil with infected dog feces or cat feces	Sometimes none; symptoms depend on what organs are involved and how extensively	Effectiveness of drug uncertain	Proper disposal of dog and cat feces, deworming of dogs

Communal infestation in school and day care settings is also common. If only a few children have pinworms, it is not necessary to screen asymptomatic children, but parents should be advised to have their children examined if symptoms (such as perianal itching) occur. Isolation of affected children is not practical, but the usual sanitation procedures—careful hand washing, proper disposal of waste, and regular disinfecting of toys and other objects that might have eggs on them—are important.

Ascariasis

The giant (up to 15 in long) intestinal roundworm (*Ascaris lumbricoides*) is occasionally found in the northern United States but is most common in the southern Appalachians, the Ozarks, and the Gulf coast states. When ascaris eggs (often present in the soil) are swallowed, they hatch in the upper intestine. The larvae penetrate the intestinal wall and travel via blood vessels and lymphatics to the lungs. They then migrate up the respiratory tree into the throat and are swallowed. Once again in the intestine, they mature to adulthood and lay eggs. These eggs, passed in the excrement, can infect the soil, setting the stage for a new reproductive cycle.

Many times infestations with these worms occur without symptoms. The most common complaint in children is abdominal pain, although pneumonia, nausea, vomiting, and weight loss may also occur. Occasionally, a worm crawls upward and is vomited or coughed up. Ascariasis is diagnosed by examining the feces (for eggs) under a microscope or by recovering a worm. Treatment consists of oral drugs (eg, Antiminth®, Vermox®, or Antepar®). In certain areas reexposure is the rule. The key to successful elimination of this parasite is sanitation.

Other Worms

Other, relatively uncommon worms are encountered periodically in certain areas. Table 16-1 summarizes pertinent facts about these parasites. Further information can be obtained from standard pediatric textbooks or from local public health authorities.

REFERENCES

Gellis SS, Kagan BM. *Current Pediatric Therapy*. 13th ed. Philadelphia, Pa: Saunders; 1990.

Oberhofer, TR. *Manual of Practical Medical Microbiology and Parasitology*. New York, NY; 1985.

Chapter 17

Lyme Disease and Infection-Related Conditions

LYME DISEASE

Lyme disease, named for Lyme, Connecticut (the location of the first major U.S. outbreak), is a multisystem disease that can affect the skin, joints, heart, and nervous system. The disorder occurs in northeastern, midwestern, and western states, and similar diseases occur in many other regions of the world, including Europe and Japan. Together, these diseases have been called borrelioses, a name derived from the causative organisms (see Color Plate 14).

Cause

Lyme disease results from infection with the tick-borne spirochete *Borrelia burgdorferi* (the spirochetes are a subset of bacteria that includes the agent that causes syphilis). Although several different tick species transmit the spirochete to humans, the deer tick (*Ixodes dammini*) accounts for most infections in the United States.

The patterns of human infection reflect the seasonal activity and distribution of infected ticks. Human disease usually begins in summer months, and the risk of Lyme disease is greater in persons who enter tick habitats (woods and fields with high grasses). Because adult ticks feed on deer, some have proposed that the increase in Lyme disease in the United States is related to rising whitetail deer populations.

Signs and Symptoms

Lyme disease usually begins 3 days to 4 weeks after the tick bite, and human disease can be divided into three stages. In stage I, the early phase of infection, skin rash predominates. The most common rash is a red dot that enlarges to form an oval or round, reddened area with a clear center (erythema migrans). Infected persons may also have fever, fatigue, muscle aches, or swollen lymph nodes during this stage. Of patients who do not receive treatment during stage I, 10% to 60% will develop new signs or symptoms that indicate spread of the spirochete to other organs or tissues.

Stage II begins a few weeks after the initial rash has resolved. Patients may experience involvement of the heart with palpitations (a sign of disturbed electrical activity of the heart) or involvement of the nervous system with aseptic meningitis, facial paralysis, or abnormalities of the nerves of the arms or legs. These neurologic complications manifest as fatigue, stiff neck, paralysis, or numbness and tingling of fingers or toes.

Complications of stage III Lyme disease may occur months to years later and typically involve the joints or the nervous system. Joint involvement (Lyme arthritis) causes pain, swelling, and redness of large joints (especially the knees) and accumulations of fluid within joints. Neurologic involvement produces various symptoms, including memory loss, mood changes, and sleep disturbances.

Diagnosis

The diagnosis of Lyme disease is suggested when a typical rash develops in a person who lives in an endemic area. Only 60% to 80% of persons infected with *B burgdorferi*, however, have characteristic rashes. Antibodies to the spirochete can be detected in the blood stream of infected persons, a fact that enables physicians to diagnose the condition in persons with other signs or symptoms compatible with Lyme disease. These antibodies usually appear 4 to 6 weeks after the onset of symptoms. Persons who live in endemic areas may have antibodies without any signs or symptoms of Lyme disease.

Management

The management of Lyme disease depends on the stage of the disorder and the presence of complications. Persons who have skin rash or facial paralysis as their only sign of Lyme disease are currently treated with antibiotic medications (eg, amoxicillin or a tetracycline) given by mouth, whereas persons with arthritis, meningitis, or other neurologic signs or symptoms require antibiotics given intravenously. It is currently debated whether early treatment with antibiotics prevents the occurrence of late signs or symptoms.

Complications

Lyme disease is not life threatening. Numerous medical complications, however, including chronic arthritis and chronic neurologic symptoms, can be part of Lyme disease. Adults with chronic disturbances of brain functions (encephalopathy) can experience forgetfulness, depression, irritability, and sleep disturbances. It is not currently known how often children with Lyme disease experience similar symptoms.

Involvement of the heart usually resolves with antibiotic therapy, and long-term heart problems are uncommon. Although treatment hastens recovery in persons with Lyme arthritis, the condition can improve gradually without medications.

Recommendations

The likelihood of acquiring Lyme disease is small, even among persons who live in endemic areas and routinely enter tick habitats. Certain precautions may reduce the likelihood of tick exposure, however. Children who play in forests or areas with high grasses should wear clothes that fit snugly around ankles, waist, and neck. The use of topical insect repellents should be considered.

Children should be examined for ticks after extended play outside, and ticks found on the children should be removed. Transmission of Lyme disease requires extended tick exposure (>24 hours), so that prompt removal of ticks probably prevents Lyme disease. The entire tick should be removed with tweezers, and the skin should be cleansed with an antiseptic such as isopropyl alcohol.

Lyme disease does not spread from person to person, so that no special precautions are necessary for children with proven or suspected Lyme disease. Rashes that are identified in children who attend child care settings should be brought to the attention of a parent who can contact the child's physician, if necessary.

RHEUMATIC FEVER

Rheumatic fever, which occurs in 1 in every 2000 children in the United States, is an inflammatory disorder that affects the heart, joints, brain, and skin.

Cause

All cases of rheumatic fever follow infection with group A streptococci. The disorder is not the direct result of bacterial infection, however. Most authorities believe that the damage to the heart and other tissues is caused instead by the antibodies that the body produces in response to these bacteria. Most cases of rheumatic fever occur in children between 5 and 15 years old, when exposure to the streptococcal bacteria is common. Certain families are affected more than others, possibly because of hereditary similarities in immune responses.

Signs and Symptoms

Most cases of rheumatic fever begin between 1 and 5 weeks after a streptococcal throat infection (which often goes undiagnosed). Signs and symptoms depend on which organs or tissues are involved. Typical features, collectively known as the Jones criteria, are painful swelling of joints (arthritis), inflammation of the heart (carditis), nodular swelling beneath the skin, jerky movements of the extremities (chorea or St Vitus' dance), and skin rash.

Pain and swelling of the joints are the most common symptoms, affecting at least 75% of children. Many children have fever as well. The heart is involved at the outset in approximately 50% of children, and about 15% have chorea. Skin rash and nodules occur less frequently. The most serious complication of rheumatic fever is damage to heart valves and muscle.

Diagnosis

There is no single laboratory test that can confirm a diagnosis of rheumatic fever, although children with this condition may have elevated blood levels of antibodies to the streptococcal bacteria (called an ASO titer), an abnormal electrocardiogram, or evidence of inflammation, indicated by an elevated blood cell sedimentation rate. In many cases, however, the diagnosis rests entirely on the presence of characteristic signs and symptoms.

Management

Once rheumatic fever begins, there is no specific therapy that can eliminate the cause. Management is directed at reducing inflammation and treating complications, particularly those involving the heart. Most children are given large amounts of aspirin for 1 to 4 weeks to reduce pain and discomfort. All children receive intramuscular penicillin to eliminate the streptococcal bacteria and thereby reduce the likelihood of recurrence or exacerbation of the disorder. Prolonged bed rest is not necessary. Most children can return to school within a few weeks, assuming that serious heart complications do not occur.

Complications

The most serious complications result from damage to the heart valves or muscle, which occurs in approximately half of children with rheumatic fever. Occasionally, children die as a result of heart failure. Others may require corrective surgical procedures, such as replacing damaged valve tissue with a mechanical valve. Children with chorea commonly have behavioral disturbances (for example, labile emotions) that may, along with the chorea, affect school performance or peer interactions. These tend to improve as the chorea subsides. Children whose only manifestation is chorea usually have the best overall prognosis.

Recommendations

Rheumatic fever itself is not a communicable disease. Group A streptococci, however, the bacteria that cause it, can be spread from child to child, usually by contact with secretions on glasses, food, and other objects that have been in the mouth. Sharing of these objects should be discouraged.

Strep throat is a common infection in children. Any child with fever, sore throat, and swollen lymph glands in the neck should be referred to a physician for diagnosis and treatment.

Children who recover from rheumatic fever may need to limit their physical activities. They should be allowed to participate in competitive sports or other strenuous activities only after a thorough examination by a physician. Such children will also require daily oral or monthly injectable penicillin for many years, possibly for life, to prevent recurrences or complications.

BOTULISM

Botulism is an uncommon and occasionally fatal neurologic disorder caused by a toxin produced by the bacterium *Clostridium botulinum*. There are two major forms of this illness: food-borne botulism, which is caused by eating toxin-containing foods; and infantile botulism, which results from intestinal infection with the bacterium itself. Between 40 and 100 cases of botulism occur in the United States each year.

Cause

Clostridium botulinum, the bacterium that produces the botulism toxin, is widespread in the human environment. It grows on many vegetable plants, and its spores are present in most soils. This organism is a relative of the bacteria that produce tetanus (*C tetani*) and gangrene (*C perfringens*).

Food-borne botulism results from eating improperly prepared foods, particularly home-canned meats or low-acid vegetables (eg, green beans, peppers, and corn), that contain the botulism toxin. This toxin is produced by contaminating spores that grow in the low-oxygen environment of sealed cans.

Infantile botulism, by contrast, occurs when infants younger than 8 months ingest the spores. Because the infant's gastrointestinal tract lacks sufficient acid to destroy the spores, they multiply and produce toxin. Soil, fruits, and honey are among several suspected sources of *C botulinum* spores.

In both types of botulism, the toxin, one of the most potent of all poisons, enters the blood stream and is carried to nerve endings, where it interferes with the transmission of acetylcholine, a chemical substance that controls autonomic and muscle functions.

Signs and Symptoms

In food-borne botulism, the incubation period typically ranges from 18 to 36 hours. The first symptoms include dry mouth, double or blurred vision, drooping eyelids, and difficulty with speech and swallowing. These symptoms are later compounded by generalized weakness of the arms, legs, and respiratory muscles (which makes breathing difficult). Only one third of patients with food-borne botulism have nausea or vomiting.

One of the earliest signs of infantile botulism is severe constipation. The affected infant sleeps more than usual and has a poor appetite. As the illness progresses, the cry and suck become weak, and the infant drools excessively. Motor tone and activity decrease, and breathing can become weak and ineffective. In severe cases, the infant may stop breathing altogether. In fact, some infants with botulism have illnesses similar to sudden infant death syndrome (crib death), a disorder that typically affects infants younger than 6 months of age.

Diagnosis

Food-borne botulism is usually suggested by the typical progression of signs and symptoms. Because the toxin interferes with neuromuscular functions, the diagnosis can usually be supported by a specialized muscle test (electromyography) and confirmed by identifying the botulism toxin in the patient's serum or feces. Any incriminated food is examined for toxin and *C botulinum* organisms.

Infantile botulism should be considered in any infant with severe constipation, a weak cry and suck, and difficulty breathing. Although toxin is rarely found in the affected infant's serum, both *C botulinum* organisms and toxin are present in the feces.

Management

Both food-borne and infantile botulism may cause illness that lasts up to several weeks. Affected individuals require intravenous fluids and close monitoring of breathing functions. Many require mechanical respirators.

Because botulism results from toxin rather than from direct infection with the bacterium, antibiotics are not useful. Food-borne botulism is sometimes treated with an antitoxin derived from the serum of horses. This antitoxin has not been proven effective, however, and it causes allergic reactions in some people. Only rarely is it used to treat cases of infantile botulism.

Complications

The vast majority of patients with food-borne or infantile botulism survive their illness. Mortality in food-borne botulism averages approximately 15%; mortality among hospitalized cases of infantile botulism is less than 5%. Some of the patients who require machine-assisted breathing for extended periods have secondary complications, such as weight loss or pneumonia.

Rarely does botulism cause long-term effects in survivors, although an occasional adult has residual symptoms, such as dry mouth or decreased endurance, that may last months or even years.

Recommendations

Food-borne botulism can be prevented by proper home canning methods. State or county extension services can provide updated recommendations regarding effective ways to reduce risk in home-canned foods. All home-canned foods, particularly meats and vegetables, should be boiled or baked before consumption. Temperatures of 180°F (80°C) or higher can inactivate the botulism toxin within 10 to 15 minutes. All suspected cases of botulism, particularly food-borne cases, should be reported promptly to local health officials.

REYE SYNDROME

Reye syndrome, a childhood disorder characterized by vomiting, disorientation, and progressive loss of consciousness, occurs in approximately 1 in every 50,000 children between the ages of 1 month and 20 years.

Cause

Reye syndrome does not result from direct infection but from infection-related injury to important cellular components of the liver, brain, and other organs. Viruses such as influenza viruses, adenoviruses, and the varicella zoster virus (the cause of chickenpox) act as triggers for Reye syndrome. Factors other than infection also contribute to the development of Reye syndrome. Several drugs, especially aspirin, have been linked to this disorder. Consequently, in 1984 the US Surgeon General recommended that aspirin therapy be avoided in young children with chickenpox and any flulike illness.

Signs and Symptoms

Reye syndrome typically begins within 3 to 10 days after the onset of a viral illness. The child starts to vomit and, within 12 to 24 hours, becomes lethargic and disoriented. Breathing is rapid (hyperventilation), and the pupils are often dilated. Thereafter, periods of agitation or combativeness may alternate with periods of coma. In most cases, the child's condition deteriorates for the first 48 to 72 hours after the onset of symptoms. In severe or untreated cases, massive brain swelling occurs, causing coma and potentially brain death. If severe complications do not occur, the child recovers rapidly during the next 2 to 4 days.

Diagnosis

Although no single laboratory test confirms the diagnosis, several abnormalities typical of this condition are revealed by laboratory tests. Most children with Reye syndrome have markedly elevated serum levels of liver-derived enzymes, such as aspartate aminotransferase; all have elevated serum ammonia levels, and many young children have low blood sugar levels. All are signs of liver damage.

Although the cerebrospinal fluid of a Reye syndrome patient is nearly always normal, a CT scan usually shows brain swelling, the most serious complication of Reye syndrome. A brain wave test (electroencephalogram) reveals abnormalities that correlate with the severity of the disorder.

Management

Management depends on the severity of the illness. In general, therapy has three goals: to treat brain swelling, to correct blood and fluid abnormalities, and to prevent complications. Mild cases can usually be treated with intravenous fluids only. In contrast, severely ill children require intensive care treatment with continuous observation of heart, lung, kidney, and brain functions.

Complications

During the earliest epidemics of Reye syndrome in Australia and the United States, as many as 50% or more of affected children died. Currently, mortality rates average 25% or less. Causes of death include shock, cardiac arrest, bleeding (the blood fails to clot because of liver damage), and brain death (caused by massive brain swelling).

Most children who survive Reye syndrome recover without major long-term disabilities. Some, however, particularly children who are severely ill or who have high blood ammonia levels, have complications such as seizures, cognitive dysfunction, and speech abnormalities.

Recommendations

Because outcome in Reye syndrome depends on early recognition and treatment, children with vomiting and altered consciousness require prompt referral to a physician. Aspirin should be avoided in children with flulike illnesses and chickenpox. Fever and pain symptoms can be treated adequately with nonaspirin drugs such as acetaminophen or ibuprofen.

Reye syndrome itself is not contagious. Illnesses that can lead to Reye syndrome, however (e.g., chickenpox or influenza), are spread from person to person in community epidemics. Good hygiene can decrease the transmission of these illnesses.

Some survivors of Reye syndrome have long-term abnormalities that affect speech, behavior, and learning. These children may benefit from formal intelligence testing and evaluation by a speech and hearing specialist. They may also require special education.

GUILLAIN-BARRÉ SYNDROME

Guillain-Barré syndrome (GBS) is a neurologic disorder that can follow several common childhood infections, including upper respiratory or gastrointestinal infections. Cases can also occur after immunization or surgery. Unlike Reye syndrome, which affects the brain, GBS affects nerves after they exit the spinal cord. GBS is not the result of direct infection of nerves but a consequence of the body's immune response to the triggering agent. Therefore, GBS is not contagious.

In most cases, the initial symptoms are pain and tingling of the hands or feet. Thereafter, patients notice muscle weakness, usually beginning in the legs and then gradually ascending to the trunk and arms. Paralysis of facial muscles may occur, causing difficulty in swallowing and speaking. The muscles of the chest may become weak, making breathing difficult and sometimes necessitating support from a mechanical respirator.

The typical case of GBS lasts from 2 to 4 weeks. Although there is no specific therapy for this disorder, children often improve when treated with intravenous immunoglobulin or when their plasma is exchanged with fresh donor plasma (a procedure known as plasmapheresis).

Approximately 5% of patients with GBS die, usually as a result of breathing difficulties or pneumonia. Two thirds of survivors recover completely. The remainder have some degree of neurologic disability, such as muscle weakness or incoordination. An occasional patient is sufficiently disabled to require a wheelchair. Because the brain is not involved, intellectual functions, hearing, and vision are not affected.

KAWASAKI DISEASE

Kawasaki disease, first described among Japanese infants, is characterized by fever lasting more than 5 days, skin rash typically involving the trunk, redness or peeling of the skin of the hands or feet, changes in the mucous membranes of the mouth (cracking or strawberry tongue), inflammation of the eyes (conjunctivitis), and swelling of lymph nodes in the neck. This disorder usually affects young children between the ages of 1 and 5 years and is uncommon in older children.

A typical case lasts 1 to 3 weeks. Fever, the first sign of the illness, is usually accompanied by Iymph node swelling and conjunctivitis. The skin rash appears during the latter half of the first week, and during the second week the skin begins to peel.

Although there is no single test that can confirm the diagnosis of Kawasaki disease, most children have abnormal white blood cell counts and prolonged red blood cell sedimentation rates, a nonspecific measure of inflammation. Some children also have elevated platelet counts.

Most children recover after 1 to 2 months without any long-term consequences. Approximately 25% have abnormalities of electrical conduction within the heart, however, and 10% to 15% develop dilatations (aneurysms) of the arteries that supply the heart with blood. These heart abnormalities cause sudden death in 1% to 2% of children with this disease. Treatment with intravenous immunoglobulin prevents long-term complications.

Kawasaki disease does not appear to be highly contagious. Affected children need not be isolated once the acute illness subsides.

The cause of Kawasaki disease has not been determined. Many investigators believe that it is the result of an infection, possibly with a virus or other small microorganism. Because the cause is not known, there is no specific treatment.

REFERENCES

Arnon SS, Chin J. Botulism. In: Wehrle PF, Top F, eds. *Communicable and Infectious Diseases.* 9th ed.St Louis, Mo: Mosby; 1981:125–134.

Bale JF Jr. Reyes syndrome. In: Rakel RE, ed. *Conn's Current Therapy.* 37th ed. Philadelphia, Pa: Saunders; 1985:751–753.

Harris JP, Washington R. Acute rheumatic fever. In: McAnarney ER, Kreipe RE, Orr DP, Comerci GD, eds. *Textbook of Adolescent Medicine.* Philadelphia, Pa: Saunders; 1992:378–381.

Kennedy RH, Danielson MA, Mulder DW, Kurland LT. Guillain-Barré syndrome: a 42-year epidemiologic and clinical study. *Mayo Clinic Proc.* 1978; 53:93–99.

Melish ME, Hicks RM, Reddy V. Kawasaki syndrome: an update. *Hosp Pract.* 1982; 17:99–106.

Rahn DW. Lyme disease: clinical manifestations, diagnosis, and treatment. *Semin Arthritis Rheum.* 1991; 20:201–218.

Ropper AH. Current concepts: the Guillain-Barré syndrome. *N Engl J Med.* 1992; 326:1130–1136.

Appendix A

Parent Handouts on Infectious Diseases

Communicating information to parents is an important part of quality child care. The following handouts, adapted from guidelines prepared by the University of Iowa Children's Health Care Center, are designed to provide frequently requested information about infectious diseases. These pages can be copied for distribution. (Copies should be prepared ahead of time to be available when needed.)

- Chickenpox
- Conjunctivitis
- Fever
- Giardiasis
- Head Lice
- *Hemophilus influenzae* infections
- Hepatitis A
- Impetigo
- Measles
- Meningitis
- Meningococcal Disease
- Mumps
- Pinworms
- Rubella
- Scabies
- Strep Throat
- Vomiting and Diarrhea
- Whooping Cough (Pertussis)

Information for Parents

Your child may have been exposed to a child with chickenpox. Please read the following information carefully.

CHICKENPOX (VARICELLA)

Chickenpox is one of the most common and most contagious viral diseases of childhood. It is caused by the varicella zoster virus and is spread through the air from secretions in the nose and throat of an infected individual or by direct contact with the skin rash. Chickenpox is most common among children under the age of 10 but can occur at any age. Occasionally, children can get chickenpox more than once. This is more likely to occur when a child first gets chickenpox at less than 1 year of age.

Signs and Symptoms

Children may begin feeling ill a day or two before the rash begins. They usually have fever and a distinctive skin rash. The rash begins as red bumps, which develop into blisters. The blister fluid is clear initially, then turns cloudy before the blisters pop and form scabs. The blisters appear in crops and may involve the entire body, including the eyes, mouth, throat, and vagina. The rash causes itching, which may be so severe that is keeps the child from sleeping. Some children have only a few blisters and some may have more than 1,000. Children with a more severe rash usually have higher fever. The fever may be as high as 104°F (40°C). If one child gets chickenpox in a family with several children, it is common for all of the nonimmune children to become infected. It is also common for the second or third cases of chickenpox in a family to be more severe than the first case.

Incubation Period: 10 to 21 days (usually 2 weeks).

Infectious Period: 1 to 2 days before the onset of the rash until 6 days after the rash develops.

Exclusion from Day Care: Children with the usual course of chickenpox may return on the sixth day after the rash begins. Children with a prolonged course should be excluded until all lesions have crusted over.

Complications

Chickenpox is usually a mild disease except in children or adults with cancer or leukemia, those taking steroids or other medications, or with other conditions that make them unable to fight infection. These individuals can develop serious illness if infected with chickenpox. If your child or someone who has been exposed to your child is at risk of severe disease, contact your physician immediately.

After infection, the varicella virus remains in the body in nerve cells and may reactivate years later resulting in shingles or herpes zoster. This is a painful, blistering rash that usually occurs in a narrow band on only one side of the body. Persons most likely to have shingles are the elderly and children who developed chickenpox in the first year of life.

Prevention and Treatment

Acetaminophen should be used for discomfort and control of fever. Aspirin has been linked to Reye syndrome (a life-threatening disease of the liver and brain) in children with chickenpox and should not be given.

Children can take antihistamines such as Benadryl or Vistaril to relieve the itching. Fingernails should be kept trimmed to decrease the trauma from scratching. Oatmeal or baking soda baths may be temporarily soothing. Sometimes the skin rash becomes infected with bacteria, resulting in impetigo, a condition that requires treatment with an antibiotic medication.

Individuals at risk of serious disease may require injection of Varicella Zoster Immune Globulin (VZIG) within 96 hours of exposure in order to prevent illness. Antiviral medication (acyclovir), if begun within the first 24 hours after onset of the rash, may decrease the number of blisters and the duration of the rash. Although available for use in normal children, this medication is most appropriate and effective in children or adults at increased risk of severe disease. The Academy of Pediatrics recommends acyclovir for children 13 and older, children with a chronic skin or lung disorder, those receiving chronic aspirin therapy, children being treated with corticosteroids, and children who are immunocompromised for some reason. A varicella vaccine may be available in the near future. Recommendations for use will be published at that time.

If you suspect chickenpox, keep your child at home and contact your physician.

If your child is diagnosed with chickenpox, tell your child care provider.

Information for Parents

Your child may have been exposed to a child with pink eye. Please read the following information carefully.

CONJUNCTIVITIS (PINK EYE)

Conjunctivitis is an inflammation (irritation) of the eyes. It can result from infection with a virus or bacterium; it can also be caused by allergies or chemicals (medication, gas fumes, chlorine from swimming pools, etc).

Infectious (viral or bacterial) conjunctivitis is contagious. It spreads from person to person by direct contact with discharge from the eyes.

Signs and Symptoms

Purulent conjunctivitis is caused by a bacterial infection. The white part of the eye and the inside of the lid become red and the child may complain of itching or pain. There is a thick white, yellow, or green discharge, and the eyelashes may be stuck together when the child awakens in the morning.

Children with purulent conjunctivitis sometimes develop an ear infection. Contact your physician if you observe any of the following signs: fever, irritability, poor sleep, loss of appetite, or tugging or hitting at the ears.

Incubation Period: Usually 2 to 7 days.

Infectious Period/Exclusion from Day Care: Until a full 24 hours after antibiotic treatment is begun.

Prevention and Treatment

Purulent conjunctivitis is treated with an antibiotic drop or ointment that is put directly into the eye. In some situations your physician may choose an antibiotic that is taken by mouth. Careful hand washing is important in preventing the spread of the disease. The child should use a separate towel from other family members. Tissues used to wipe the pus from the eyes should be disposed of carefully and the caregiver should wash his or her hands immediately afterward.

If you suspect purulent conjunctivitis, keep your child at home and contact your physician. If your child has conjunctivitis, tell your child care provider.

Information for Parents

FEVER

The normal body temperature is approximately 98.6°F (37.0°C), but it can range between 97.0°F (36.1°C) and 100.4°F (38.0°C). Fever is usually considered present if the child has:

- a rectal temperature above 100.4°F (38.0°C)
- an oral temperature above 100.0°F (37.8°C)
- an axillary temperature above 99.0°F (37.2°C)

Generally speaking, fever is not harmful until it reaches approximately 106°F (41.1°C).

Treatment

Dress the child in lightweight clothing to allow heat loss through the skin. Give antifever medication only if the child is uncomfortable or the fever is very high. Acetaminophen can be given every 4 hours (up to five doses in a 24-hour period) (Tables A-1 and A-2). Acetaminophen (Tylenol®, Tempra®, Liquiprin®, Panadol®, etc) is preferred for infants and children. Aspirin may be given to older children unless they have certain viral illnesses, such as chickenpox or influenza. Consult your physician before giving aspirin if you suspect that your child has a viral illness.

Ibuprofen liquid is also available by prescription for fever control in children. Contact your physician for more information.

Always consult your physician before administering medication to children younger than 2 years.

When To Seek Medical Attention

Immediate medical attention is required if the child has a fever and any of the following:

- is younger than 2 months
- has a temperature higher than 105°F (40.6°C)
- is difficult to awaken
- is confused or delirious

Table A-1 Recommended Acetaminophen Dosage

Child's Age	*Child's weight (pounds)*	*Drug dose*
	Acetaminophen*	
0–3 months	6-11	40 mg
4–11 months	12–17	80 mg
12–24 months	18–23	120 mg
2–3 years	24–35	160 mg
4–5 years	36–47	240 mg
6–8 years	48–59	320 mg
9–10 years	60–71	400 mg
11–12 years	72–95	480 mg
12 years and older	96 and over	325–650 mg

KEEP ALL MEDICINES IN A LOCKED CABINET—OUT OF REACH OF SMALL CHILDREN.

- is crying inconsolably
- is acting very sick
- is considered at high risk for a serious infection (ie, has an immune deficiency disease, sickle cell disease, or is taking medication that impairs the immune system)
- has a seizure
- has a stiff neck
- has purple or red spots on the skin that do not temporarily disappear when pressed with a finger
- has difficulty breathing (rapid, labored, or hard breathing) that does not improve when the nose is cleared

Table A-2 Acetaminophen Preparations

Type	*Concentration*
Infant drops	80 mg per 0.8 cc
Syrup (elixir)	160 mg per 5 cc
Chewable tablets	80 mg each or 160 mg each
Junior-strength swallow tablets	160 mg each
Regular tablets	320 mg each

Always read the package instructions carefully before administration.

Less urgent but prompt medical attention is necessary if the child has a fever and any of the following:

- is 2 to 4 months old
- has a temperature of 104°F (40°C), especially if the child is younger than 2 years
- has burning or pain with urination
- has ear pain
- walks with a limp that was not present previously
- complains of abdominal pain
- has fever for more than 72 hours
- has fever for more than 24 hours without obvious cause or location of infection
- has fever that ceases for more than 24 hours then recurs

Information for Parents

Your child may have been exposed to a child with giardiasis. Please read the following information carefully.

GIARDIASIS

Giardia lamblia is a parasite that commonly causes an intestinal infection in children and adults. It is spread by feces or contaminated food or water. Infected animals (eg, dogs and beavers) can also pass *Giardia* parasites along to humans. In day care centers infection is often spread by contaminated hands (children's or caretakers'), toys, furniture, carpets, or wading pools.

Signs and Symptoms

Sometimes giardiasis occurs without symptoms. At other times it causes diarrhea (which may alternate with constipation). Infected children may also have excessive gas, abdominal bloating, poor appetite, and weight loss. Young children may have vomiting.

Incubation Period: 1 to 4 weeks.

Infectious Period: Children are contagious (able to spread the infection) as long as they shed the parasite cysts in their stools.

Exclusion from Day Care: Infected children or staff with symptoms should be kept out of day care until they have been treated and no longer have diarrhea. Infected individuals without symptoms have little risk of spreading the infection and usually do not require treatment or exclusion.

Prevention and Treatment

If an outbreak of giardiasis is suspected in a day care center, the health department should be contacted to assist with management. All children and staff who have symptoms (ie, diarrhea, vomiting, etc) should be screened for infection. Stools may be examined under the microscope for evidence of the parasite. It may be necessary to examine several different stool samples collected over a week or two to be sure that the child is not infected. Some communities may have access to a rapid detection method for giardiasis that provides immediate results. Following this screening procedure, the health department will make recommendations for treatment and prevention of spread.

Several different medications are available for treating giardiasis infections. Contact your physician if you suspect that you or your child has giardiasis or if you have further questions.

Information for Parents

Your child may have been exposed to a child with head lice. Please read the following information carefully.

HEAD LICE

Lice are wingless, insectlike parasites that live on the hairy parts of the body. They are often found in schools, day care centers, and other crowded settings where children are in close contact. Lice are transmitted by direct contact with an infected child or adult or, indirectly, by sharing hats, scarves, brushes, or barrettes. They cannot jump or fly.

The female louse deposits her eggs (nits) on the hair near the scalp. These nits appear as white-gray grains stuck to the hair shaft. Nits and lice can usually be found near the nape of the neck or behind the ears and can be seen with the naked eye, although a magnifying glass can be helpful. Adult lice are darker colored and may be seen moving through the hair. With severe infestations itching of the scalp can be intense.

Infectious Period/Exclusion from Day Care: Infected children should be excluded from day care until the morning after treatment.

Prevention and Treatment

Good personal hygiene and careful grooming cannot protect your child from lice. If head lice infestation occurs, it can be treated with a prescription or a nonprescription pediculicide (such as Kwell®, Nix®, Rid®, etc).

Some products require a second treatment; others are effective with a single treatment. Some physicians may recommend a second treatment 1 week after the first regardless of the pediculicide used. Toxicity may occur with misuse; follow package or prescription directions carefully. Permethrin may persist on the hair for 2 weeks or more, making reinfection less likely during this period. Clothing or bedding can be disinfected by machine washing and drying. Articles that cannot be washed can be dry cleaned or stored in a sealed plastic bag for at least 10 days. Brushes or combs should be washed with a pediculicide. Mattresses, furniture, and rugs should be vacuumed.

Some schools have "no nit" policies requiring children to be nit-free before returning to day care or school. This has not been proven to be necessary to interrupt transmission but may be a way to ensure that children have been treated. Nit removal may be facilitated by a vinegar and water solution applied to the hair to loosen the nits and use of a specially designed, fine-tooth comb.

Check your child for nits and lice daily for the next 2 weeks. If you think your child is infected, contact your health care provider for recommendations. If your child is diagnosed with head lice, contact your child care provider.

Information for Parents

Your child may have been exposed to a child with Hemophilus influenzae *type B disease. Please read the following information carefully.*

HEMOPHILUS INFLUENZAE INFECTIONS

The bacterium *Hemophilus influenzae* type b is one of the most common causes of meningitis in children younger than 5 years. Children exposed to this bacterium can develop any one of a number of diseases (Table A-3).

Treatment

Antibiotics are effective in treating diseases due to *Hemophilus influenzae* type b. For the best outcome, treatment should begin as soon as infection is suspected.

Table A-3 Infections Caused by *Hemophilus influenzae* type b

Infection	*Description*	*Possible signs and symptoms*
Meningitis	Infection of the membranes that cover the brain and spinal cord	High fever, irritability, extreme sleepiness, restlessness, poor appetite, headache, or stiff neck
Bacteremia	Infection of the blood stream	Ill appearance, high fever, fatigue, irritability
Epiglottitis	Infection of the epiglottis and other structures deep within the throat; swelling blocks airways, causing death unless emergency medical treatment is given	Anxious appearance and apparent air hunger; high-pitched, crowing noises, and leaning forward to breathe more easily
Cellulitis	Infection of the skin	Area of skin (usually around the eye or cheek) is swollen, warm, tender, and red or purple; high fever and ill appearance
Pneumonia	Infection of the lungs	Fever, cough, and difficulty breathing
Septic arthritis	Infection of a joint (often the hip joint)	Fever and a limp that was not present previously

Incubation Period: Unknown, variable.

Infectious Period/Exclusion from Day Care: Infected children should be excluded until a physician determines that reentry is safe.

Prevention

A vaccine is available to prevent *Hemophilus influenzae* type b disease. This series of immunizations is begun at 2 months of age and is recommended for all infants.

The antibiotic rifampin is sometimes indicated for contacts of infected children to prevent the spread of *Hemophilus influenzae* disease in day care. The local health department has been contacted for recommendations. In the event that rifampin prophylaxis is recommended, you will be notified by an attachment to this notice. If rifampin is recommended, all children and staff in the classroom of the exposed child (regardless of immunization status) should receive the antibiotic promptly in order to reduce the chance of spread.

During the next month, particularly during the next week, observe your child carefully for any signs of illness or fever and report these to your physician immediately. If your child is diagnosed with *Hemophilus influenzae* disease, please contact your child care provider. If you have further questions, please contact your physician.

Information for Parents

Your child may have been exposed to a child with hepatitis A infection. Please read the following information carefully.

HEPATITIS A

Hepatitis A is a viral infection of the liver. It is usually passed from hand to mouth after contact with the feces of an infected person. It can also be passed by contaminated food or water.

Signs and Symptoms

Infants and young children often have no symptoms. The likelihood of having jaundice—a yellowish tint to the skin and eyes—increases with age (most young children do not have it; most adults do). Other symptoms in children or adults may include loss of appetite, fatigue, nausea, vomiting, muscle aches, fever, dark urine, and pale, clay-colored stools.

Incubation Period: usually between 15 and 50 days.

Infectious Period: Individuals are probably contagious from approximately 2 weeks prior to the onset of symptoms until approximately 1 week after jaundice is first noted.

Exclusion from Day Care: Children or day care staff with hepatitis A should be excluded until 1 week after the onset of symptoms and until jaundice has resolved.

Prevention and Treatment

Although no effective treatment for hepatitis A is available, most children and adults recover completely.

Good personal and environmental hygiene is important to prevent the spread of hepatitis A. Always wash your hands thoroughly before preparing food and after using the toilet or changing a diaper. In certain situations, an injection of immunoglobulin may be given to exposed children and adults to prevent spread of the virus. Immunoglobulin is a blood product that contains antibodies. The local health department will be involved in the evaluation and management of this disease. They will decide whether immunoglobulin should be given and who should receive it.

If hepatitis A infection occurs in your child's day care center, the center is likely to remain open. Moving your child to another day care center is not recommended, because this could cause further spread of the infection.

If your child or anyone in your family develops symptoms of hepatitis A infection, contact your physician or local health department. Also notify your day care center at once to protect other children and their families.

Information for Parents

Your child may have been exposed to a child with impetigo. Please read the following information carefully.

IMPETIGO

Impetigo is a common skin infection in young children. It occurs when bacteria invade skin that is broken, irritated, scratched, or burned. The areas most often affected are the hands and face, especially around the nose and mouth. Frequent sites of infection include noses that are picked, lips that are licked, thumbs that are sucked, or insect bites that are scratched.

Impetigo is contagious and can be spread—by the hands or direct contact with the lesions—to different parts of the body or to other children. The infection can also be spread by clothes or towels that have been contaminated by open sores.

Signs and Symptoms

Impetigo usually begins as red spots, which fill with fluid (blisters). The blisters rupture easily, and the fluid dries and forms a honey-colored crust. Sometimes the blisters do not rupture, or they rupture without forming crusts, producing a raw, reddened area instead.

Impetigo does not cause fever.

Incubation Period: 4 to 10 days.

Infectious Period/Exclusion from Day Care: Children should be excluded from day care until 24 hours after antibiotic treatment is begun.

Treatment

Impetigo may be treated with an antibiotic ointment, antibiotics that are taken by mouth, or both. When applying an ointment, first remove the crusts with gentle washing or soaking.

To prevent spread, make sure that persons who have contact with the sores wash their hands well with soap and water. Affected children should have their own washcloths and towels.

If you suspect impetigo, keep your child at home and contact your physician. If your child is diagnosed with impetigo, contact your child care provider.

Information for Parents

Your child may have been exposed to a child with measles. Please read the following information carefully.

MEASLES

Measles (also called rubeola and red or hard measles) is a serious viral disease of childhood. It is spread by mucous secretions from the nose and mouth.

Signs and Symptoms

Symptoms usually appear 10 days after exposure to the virus. They include high fever, cough, coldlike symptoms, conjunctivitis (inflammation of the eyes), and a red, blotchy rash that begins on the neck and spreads downward to cover the entire body.

Possible complications include ear infections, pneumonia, and, in rare cases, inflammation of the brain (encephalitis).

Incubation Period: 8 to 12 days.

Infectious Period: Children are usually infectious from 1 to 2 days prior to the onset of any symptoms or 3 to 5 days prior to development of the rash until 4 days after the rash appears.

Exclusion from Day Care: Children should be excluded until 6 days after the onset of rash.

Prevention

Measles is a vaccine-preventable disease. The Advisory Committee on Immunization Practices recommends that all children be immunized against measles, mumps, and rubella (MMR) at 15 months of age. Children who are vaccinated before 12 months of age should be reimmunized at 15 months. People born before 1957 are usually immune as a result of past infection. A second dose of MMR is recommended before school entry (4 to 6 years of age) or at entry into middle school (11 to 12 years of age). If your child has not been immunized, contact your health care provider.

If your child develops any symptoms of this disease, contact your physician. If your child is diagnosed with measles, contact your child care provider.

Information for Parents

Your child may have been exposed to a child with meningitis. Please read the following information carefully.

MENINGITIS

Meningitis is an inflammation of the membranes that cover the brain and spinal cord. It can be caused by viruses or bacteria. Although viral meningitis is generally mild, bacterial meningitis is a serious infection that can be fatal without prompt antibiotic treatment.

Signs and Symptoms

Meningitis can cause high fever, severe headache, stiff neck, extreme fussiness or sleepiness, poor feeding, failure to respond to the environment, or an unwillingness to be cuddled and held.

Diagnosis

To diagnose meningitis, the physician inserts a needle into the spine and withdraws some of the fluid (this is called a spinal tap). The fluid is examined under a microscope for pus cells and bacteria. The fluid is also cultured to identify the bacteria (if any are present).

Prevention

One of the most common causes of bacterial meningitis among children younger than 5 years of age is *Hemophilus influenzae* type b. Infection with this bacterium can be prevented by a vaccine. *Neisseria meningitidis* (meningococcus) is another common cause of bacterial meningitis. Certain types of meningitis can be prevented by administering specific antibiotics to exposed individuals. If your child has symptoms of meningitis, contact your physician immediately. If your child is diagnosed with meningitis, contact your child care provider.

Information for Parents

Your child may have been exposed to a child or staff with meningococcal disease. Please read the following information carefully.

MENINGOCOCCAL DISEASE (*NEISSERIA MENINGITIDIS*)

Signs and Symptoms

The meningococcus most commonly causes infection of the blood stream (meningococcemia) with fever, chills, and a rash characterized by bleeding into the skin. Without treatment, shock, coma, and death can follow rapidly. Meningococcus also causes meningitis with fever, headache, stiff neck, extreme lethargy or fussiness, and poor feeding. Meningococcal disease can also be complicated by infection of the joints or other parts of the body.

Incubation Period: 1 to 10 days

Infectious Period: Until 24 hours after antibiotics are begun.

Exclusion from Day Care: The infected child must be excluded from day care until the local health department or the child's physician determines that reentry is safe.

Prevention and Treatment

Prevention of disease by prophylaxis with the antibiotic rifampin is recommended for day care contacts of individuals infected with *Neisseria meningitidis*. This antibiotic will help eliminate the meningococcal organism from the nose and throat of exposed individuals and thus prevent the spread of disease. When recommended by the local health department, rifampin should be administered to all contacts within 24 hours of diagnosis of the index case (the first case of disease).

If rifampin is recommended, all children should be excluded from the center or home until after the first dose of rifampin has been administered.

Your child care provider has notified the local health department and will instruct you as to whether the antibiotic rifampin will be provided by the health department or should be obtained from your child's health care provider.

Oberve your child closely for the next month. If your child becomes ill or develops a fever, contact a physician immediately. If your child is diagnosed with meningococcal disease, contact your child care provider.

Information for Parents

Your child may have been exposed to a child with mumps. Please read the following information carefully.

MUMPS

Mumps is a viral disease of childhood. It is spread from person to person by respiratory secretions (mucus from the nose or mouth).

Signs and Symptoms

Signs and symptoms of mumps include fever, headache, and swelling and tenderness of the glands located at the angle of the jaw (just in front of and below the ears). Mumps can cause inflammation of the testes in postpubertal boys. Other possible complications of this disease include hearing loss and inflammation of the brain and its membranes (meningoencephalitis).

Incubation Period: 12 to 25 days after exposure.

Infectious Period: Children are usually infectious from 7 days before the onset of gland swelling until 9 days after swelling appears.

Exclusion from Day Care: Infected children should be excluded until 9 days after parotid gland swelling was noted.

Prevention

Mumps is a vaccine-preventable disease. The Advisory Committee on Immunization Practices recommends that all children be immunized at 15 months of age with the measles, mumps and rubella vaccines (MMR). A second dose is given prior to school entry (4 to 6 years of age) or at entry into middle school (11 to 12 years of age).

If your child has not been immunized against mumps, contact your physician or public health agency to arrange for vaccination. If you suspect mumps, keep your child at home and contact your physician. If your child is diagnosed with mumps, contact your child care provider.

Information for Parents

Your child may have been exposed to a child with pinworms. Please read the following information carefully.

PINWORMS

Pinworms are small (less than 1/2 in long), white, threadlike worms that commonly infest the intestines. They are easily spread from person to person by contact with feces that contain the eggs. The eggs can be carried on the hands, clothing, bedding, food, and so forth. Pinworms cannot be passed from animals to humans. Pinworms are particularly common among children in schools and day care centers.

Signs and Symptoms

Infection is usually characterized by intense rectal itching, which is often worse at night, when the female worms crawl out of the rectum to lay their eggs. These worms may also infect the vagina, causing itching and irritation.

Often, the worms can be seen by inspecting the child's rectal area during sleep. Diagnosis can also be made by placing clear cellophane tape on the anus as soon as the child awakens in the morning and having your physician examine this tape under the microscope for eggs.

Prevention and Treatment

If you suspect that your child has pinworms, call your physician. There are several medications that can be used to effectively treat pinworm infestation. When a child has pinworms, many physicians recommend that all family members receive treatment at the same time.

To prevent reinfection, wash bedding and clothing in hot water. Also, instruct your children always to wash their hands after using the toilet and before eating. Despite such measures, however, reinfection is common.

Information for Parents

Your child may have been exposed to a child with rubella. Please read the following information carefully.

RUBELLA

Rubella (German measles) is a viral disease of childhood. It is spread by respiratory secretions (mucus from the nose and mouth), blood, or urine from an infected person.

When an unimmunized pregnant woman becomes infected with rubella, her child can die before birth or can be born with serious birth defects, such as cataracts, mental retardation, deafness, heart defects, skin rash, and enlargement of the liver and spleen.

Signs and Symptoms

Children with rubella usually have a mild fever; a red, bumpy rash; and large, tender lymph nodes behind the ear and at the back of the head and neck.

Adults may have low fever, headache, and runny nose. They may also have pain and swelling of the joints (arthritis or arthralgia). Infection may also occur without obvious symptoms. In rare cases, inflammation of the brain (encephalitis) occurs.

Incubation Period: 14 to 21 days after exposure.

Infectious Period:

- Postnatal rubella: from approximately 1 week before the rash until 7 days afterward.
- Congenital rubella: congenitally infected infants should be considered contagious until 1 year of age or until rubella cultures of urine and nasopharyngeal secretions (obtained after 3 months of age) are negative.

Exclusion from Day Care:

- Postnatal rubella: until 7 days after onset of rash.
- Congenital rubella: until 1 year of age or until urine and nasopharyngeal cultures are negative.

Prevention

Rubella is a highly contagious disease that can be prevented by vaccination. The Advisory Committee on Immunization Practices recommends that all children are immunized against measles, mumps, and rubella at 15 months of age.

A second dose of vaccine should be given prior to school entry (4 to 6 years of age) or at entry into middle school (11 to 12 years of age).

If your child has not been immunized against rubella, contact your physician or public health agency to arrange for a vaccination. If you suspect rubella infection, keep your child at home and contact your physician. If your child is diagnosed with rubella, contact your child care provider.

Information for Parents

Your child may have been exposed to a child with scabies. Please read the following information carefully.

SCABIES

Scabies is a common infestation of the skin caused by the itch mite. This parasite is spread by close contact with the skin, clothing, or bedding of an infected person. Symptoms may appear any time from several days to several weeks after contact.

Signs and Symptoms

Scabies causes severe itching, which is often most intense at night (it can awaken the child). Infants are usually affected on the palms, soles, head, neck, and face. Adults and older children are generally affected on the hands, wrists, elbows, buttocks, and genitals, and between the fingers and toes.

Affected skin may have tiny burrows (these look like raised lines or scratches), bumps, blisters, or scaly patches. In other cases, the skin looks as if it has been severely scratched and is raw and bleeding.

Incubation Period: First infection, 4 to 6 weeks after exposure. With repeat infections, symptoms develop within 1 to 4 days.

Exclusion from Day Care: The child can return to day care the day after treatment is completed.

Treatment

If you suspect that your child has scabies, see your physician. If scabies is diagnosed, your physician will prescribe a medication that you can apply to kill the mites. Usually, all family members are treated.

Wash or dry clean all clothing and bedding, since the mite can live away from humans for 2 to 3 days.

Even after treatment, the itching may persist for weeks after the mites have been killed because of sensitivity to the mite or mite feces. Ask your physician about a medication to help reduce the itching.

Information for Parents

Your child may have been exposed to a child with strep throat. Please read the following information carefully.

STREP THROAT

Strep throat and scarlet fever (strep throat with a rash) are caused by the bacterium group A streptococcus. This organism is spread by contact with secretions from the mouth and nose of infected persons.

Signs and Symptoms

Signs and symptoms include sore throat, fever, swollen glands below the jaw and in the neck, and pus on the tonsils. Sometimes there is a fine, red, sandpapery rash. Vomiting and stomach pain may also occur.

Incubation Period: 2 to 4 days after exposure.

Exclusion from Day Care: Infected children should be excluded until 24 hours after antibiotics are started.

Treatment

If you suspect strep throat, keep your child at home and contact your physician, who will perform a throat culture to determine whether the streptococcal bacterium is present. Children exposed to strep throat usually do not require a throat culture unless they develop symptoms.

If your child is diagnosed with strep throat, he/she will be given an antibiotic injection or a prescription for an antibiotic to be taken by mouth. To prevent more serious disease (such as rheumatic fever), your child must take this medication as prescribed for a full 10 days, even if the symptoms are gone and your child is feeling well.

If your child is diagnosed with strep throat, contact your child care provider.

Information for Parents

Your child may have been exposed to a child with vomiting and diarrhea. Please read the following information carefully.

VOMITING AND DIARRHEA

Most illnesses with vomiting and diarrhea are mild and respond well to simple therapy.

Treatment

For diarrhea, begin encouraging liquids right away. With this disorder, the amount of liquids consumed is more important than the amount of solid foods. The best fluid to offer is an oral electrolyte solution (such as Pedialyte®, Ricelyte®, or Rehydralyte®) specially formulated for infants and young children. Do not use fluids such as Gatorade, fruit juice, or soft drinks, particularly with young infants. Older infants and children taking solids can continue to be offered a regular diet as recommended by your health care provider. Bananas, rice, cooked cereal, applesauce, noodles, and cooked meat are good choices. Unless otherwise instructed by your physician, breastfeeding or formula should be continued. Clear liquids should be offered between feedings.

If your child has vomited, continue to give the electrolyte solution in very small amounts; a teaspoon every few minutes. Gradually increase amounts offered as tolerated.

Signs of Trouble

A danger of severe or prolonged diarrhea and/or vomiting is dehydration—a loss of the body's normal water content. A young infant can become severely dehydrated rapidly. Signs of dehydration include:

- extreme thirst
- decreased frequency and/or amount of urination (most infants have 6 or more wet diapers per day)
- lethargy and listlessness
- sunken eyes, dry lips and mouth, absence of tears
- skin that feels doughy or does not snap back when pinched

Diarrhea and/or vomiting can accompany ear infections, urinary tract infections, or other problems that require medical attention. Contact your physician if any of the following occurs:

- The diarrhea and vomiting do not respond to therapy.
- Your child has signs of dehydration, ear infection, or bladder infection.
- There is bloody diarrhea, persistent high fever, or extreme irritability.

Information for Parents

Your child may have been exposed to a child with whooping cough. Please read the following information carefully.

WHOOPING COUGH (PERTUSSIS)

Whooping cough is a serious and sometimes fatal disease of infancy and childhood. It can lead to pneumonia, convulsions, coma, and death, particularly in infants younger than 1 year of age.

Whooping cough is caused by the bacterium *Bordetella pertussis* and is passed from person to person by respiratory secretions.

Signs and Symptoms

Initial symptoms include sneezing, runny nose, and cough. Fever is usually absent or mild. After a week or two, the child has sudden, violent attacks of coughing (paroxysms), which may be accompanied by a high-pitched whoop, or crowing noise. These coughing spells may be followed by vomiting of mucus. Between bouts of coughing, the child usually appears well.

Incubation Period: 6 to 20 days.

Infectious Period: Infected children are contagious for as long as 3 weeks after the onset of the paroxysmal cough, or for 5 days after treatment with erythromycin has begun.

Exclusion from Day Care: Infected children should be excluded from day care until 5 days after erythromycin is begun.

Prevention and Treatment

Whooping cough is contagious. The antibiotic erythromycin can stop the spread of the disease and, if given early, may even help shorten the duration of illness.

Whooping cough can be prevented by immunization. The National Advisory Committee on Immunization Practices recommends immunizing children against pertussis, tetanus, and diphtheria (DTP) beginning at 6 to 8 weeks of age.

If a case of whooping cough occurs at your child's school or day care center, a booster shot of DTP should be given to any unimmunized or inadequately immunized children younger than 7 years who have not received at least 4 doses of DTP, and children younger than 7 years who have not received a DTP vaccine within the last 3 years (according to recommended DTP/DTaP immunization schedule). Other household or day care contacts may also require vaccination.

Your physician may wish to give erythromycin to prevent infection of certain exposed individuals. Contact your physician to discuss this recommendation.

If your child has not been immunized against pertussis, arrange for a vaccination as soon as possible. If your child has been exposed to pertussis and develops any symptoms of this disease, keep the child at home and contact your physician. If your child is diagnosed with pertussis, contact your child care provider.

Appendix B

Proper Hand Washing Techniques

Use soap and warm running water. Rub hands vigorously for at least 10 seconds. Wash all skin surfaces, including:

- backs of hands
- wrists
- between fingers
- under fingernails

Rinse well under warm running water. Dry hands with a disposable towel. Turn off water with a disposable towel, not with bare hands.

Appendix C

Proper Diapering Technique

1. CHECK to be sure all necessary supplies are ready.
2. PLACE roll paper or disposable towel on diapering surface.
3. LAY the child on the diapering surface, taking care that the soiled diaper touches only your hands—not your arms or clothing.
4. REMOVE the soiled diaper and clothing.
   - Put disposable diapers in a plastic bag or plastic-lined receptacle.
   - Put soiled clothes in a plastic bag to be taken home.
5. CLEAN the child's bottom with a premoistened disposable towelette or a damp paper towel.
   - Dispose of the towelette or paper towel in the plastic bag or plastic-lined receptacle.
   - Remove the paper towel from beneath the child and dispose of it the same way.
6. WIPE your hands with a premoistened towelette or a damp paper towel.
   - Dispose of this towel in the plastic bag or plastic-lined receptacle.
7. DIAPER or dress the child. Now you can hold the child close to you.
8. WASH the child's hands and return the child to the crib or group.
9. CLEAN and DISINFECT the diapering area and any equipment and supplies you touched.
10. WASH your hands.

Note: Disposable gloves should be worn by the caregiver during diapering in case of severe dermatitis or hand abrasions with open sores. Gloves should also be worn if the infant has severe dermatitis requiring care (ie, diaper dermatitis) or if there is a risk of exposure to blood or body fluids containing blood. Gloves are not a substitution for handwashing. If gloves are worn, they should be removed carefully to avoid skin contact with the soiled glove surface. Hands should be washed as described after gloves are removed.

Source: Adapted from Centers for Disease Control. "What You Can Do To Stop Disease in Child Day Care Centers." Atlanta: Department of Health and Human Services, 1985. To be copied and displayed at the diaper changing station.

Appendix D

Additional Resources

American Public Health Association and American Academy of Pediatrics. *Caring for OurChildren: National Health and Safety Performance Standards and Guidelines for Out-of-Home Child Care Programs.* Available from the American Public Health Association, 1015 18th Street, N.W., Washington, DC 20036, or from the American Academy of Pediatrics, 141 Northwest Point Boulevard, P.O. Box 927, Elk Grove Village, IL 60009-0927.

Beneson A, ed. *Control of Communicable Diseases in Man.* 15th ed. Washington: American Public Health Association; 1990. Available from the American Public Health Association, 1015 18th Street, N.W., Washington, DC 20036.

Berezin J, ed. *The Complete Guide to Choosing Child Care.* New York: Random House; 1990.

Brown AK, Fielding JE, McKay RJ, eds. Pediatrics and child care: Papers from a Johnson & Johnson Pediatric Institute symposium "Day Care for Children." *Pediatrics.* 1993;91:1

Canadian Paediatric Society. *Well Beings: A Guide to Promote the Physical Health, Safety, and Emotional Well-Being of Children in Child Care Centres and Family Day Care Homes.* 2 vols. Available from the Canadian Paediatric Society, 401 Smyth Road, Ottawa, Ontario K1H 8L1, Canada.

Centers for Disease Control. *Morbidity and Mortality Weekly Report.* Subscription information available from the Centers for Disease Control, 1600 Clifton Road, Atlanta, GA 30333.

Centers for Disease Control. *What You Can Do To Stop Disease in Child Day Care Centers.* Atlanta: Centers for Disease Control, U.S. Department of Health and Human Services, 1985. Available from local health departments or from Public Health Advisor, Center for Professional Development and Training, Centers for Disease Control, 1600 Clifton Road, Atlanta, GA 30333.

Committee on Early Childhood, Adoption, & Dependent Care: *Health in Day Care: A Manual for Health Professionals.* Elk Grove Village, Ill. American Academy of Pediatrics; 1987. Available from the American Academy of Pediatrics, 141 Northwest Point Boulevard, P.O. Box 927, Elk Grove Village, IL 60009-0927.

Committee on School Health Staff. *School Health: A Guide for Health Professionals.* Elk Grove Village, Ill. American Academy of Pediatrics; 1987. Available from the American Academy of Pediatrics, 141 Northwest Point Boulevard, P.O. Box 927, Elk Grove Village, IL 60009-0927.

Gunzenhauser M and Caldwell BM, eds. *Group Care for Young Children.* Skillman, NJ: Johnson & Johnson Baby Products. Available from Johnson & Johnson Baby Products Company, Grandview Road, Skillman, NJ 08558.

Hein K et al, eds. *AIDS: Trading Fears for Facts. A Guide for Young People.* Fairfield, OH: Consumer Reports Books. Available from Consumer Reports Books, 9180 Le Saint Drive, Fairfield, OH 45014-5452.

Kendrick AS, Kaufmann R, and Messenger KP, eds. *Healthy Young Children: A Manual for Programs.* Washington: National Association for the Education of Young Children. Available from the National Association for the Education of Young Children, 1834 Connecticut Avenue, N.W., Washington, DC 20009-5786.

Murphy T. Infection related to day-care attendance. *Pediatric Annals* 20(8), 1991.

United States Department of Labor. *Occupational Exposure to Bloodborne Pathogens.* Available from the United States Department of Labor, Occupational Safety and Health Administration.

Glossary

A

Abscess: A localized, walled-off area of bacterial, parasitic, or fungal infection.

Acquired Immunodeficiency Syndrome (AIDS): A life-threatening illness in which the body defense mechanisms against infection and cancer fail. Caused by a virus (human immunodeficiency virus type 1 [HIV-1]) that infects cells of the human immune system.

Acyclovir: An antiviral drug used to treat herpes simplex and varicella zoster virus infections.

Adhesive Otitis: Scarring of the middle ear caused by chronic ear infections.

Aerobe: A bacterium that requires oxygen for growth.

Alopecia: Loss of hair.

Amebiasis: A disorder with vomiting and diarrhea. Caused by the protozoan *Entamoeba histolytica*.

Amoxicillin: An antibiotic of the penicillin group. Commonly used to treat ear infections in children.

Amphotericin B: A medication used to treat fungal infections.

Ampicillin: An antibiotic of the penicillin group. Commonly used to treat many childhood infections, including otitis media, meningitis, and pneumonia.

Anaerobe: A bacterium that grows in the absence of oxygen.

Analgesic: A drug used to control pain.

Anaphylaxis: An acute life-threatening allergic reaction.

Anthrax: Infection with the microorganism *Bacillus anthracis*. Usually associated with skin infection, although invasive disease can occur.

Antibody: A molecule produced by the body in response to a foreign substance, such as a virus or bacterium.

Anticonvulsant: A medication used to control seizures. Commonly used drugs include phenytoin (Dilantin®), phenobarbital, carbamazepine (Tegretol®), and valproic acid (Depakene®).

Antigen: A substance that triggers an immune response.

Antihistamine: A medication that counteracts the effects of histamine, a body chemical responsible for many allergy symptoms.

Antipyretic: A medication used to control fever.

Antitoxin: A serum or antibody that neutralizes a toxin.

Antiviral Agent: A drug that kills or inhibits the growth of viruses.

Aqueductal Stenosis: Blockage of the outflow of cerebrospinal fluid within the brain. A potential complication of congenital infections or bacterial meningitis.

Arboviruses: A group of viruses spread by insects (arthropods).

Arthritis: Infection or inflammation of the joints.

Ascariasis: An illness caused by the parasite *Ascaris lumbricoides* (a roundworm).

Aseptic: Literally, "without bacteria." A term used to describe disorders not caused by bacteria.

Asthma: A chronic, noninfectious disorder characterized by repeated episodes of wheezing, cough, and difficulty in breathing.

Ataxia: Loss of motor coordination.

Audiometry: Hearing test. Usually of two types: behavioral, in which the ability to hear is determined by the child's behavior; and brain-stem evoked, in which hearing is tested by the electrical response of the brain to sounds.

AZT (Azidothymidine or Zidovudine): An antiviral drug used to treat patients infected with HIV, the cause of AIDS.

B

Bacillary Dysentery: Severe vomiting and diarrhea caused by shigella bacteria that infect the stomach and intestines.

Bacterium: A microorganism, smaller than a human cell, that has a cell wall and contains genetic material.

Bacteriuria: The presence of bacteria in the urine.

Borrelia burgdorferi: The spirochete that causes Lyme disease.

Botulism: A neurologic and gastrointestinal disorder. Caused by a toxin that is produced by the bacterium *Clostridium botulinum*.

Bronchiolitis: Infection or inflammation of the small air passages of the lung.

Bronchitis: Infection or inflammation of the large-walled air passages of the lung.

Brucellosis: An illness associated with fever, chills, muscle aches, and loss of appetite due to *Brucella* bacteria.

C

Campylobacter: A genus of bacteria that can produce diarrhea in children.

Candidiasis: A yeast (*Candida albicans*) infection of the mouth and diaper area. Can cause serious infections in patients with abnormal immune systems.

Cat Scratch Disease: An illness caused by a bacterium and characterized by swollen lymph nodes. Associated with contact with cats.

Cellulitis: Infection of the skin or tissue beneath the skin.

Cephalosporin: An antibiotic family that comprises cefaclor, cefotaxime, ceftriaxone, and many others.

Chagas Disease: An illness due to infection with the protozoan *Trypanosoma cruzi.*

Chickenpox: An illness characterized by fever and rash. Caused by the varicella-zoster virus, the same virus that causes shingles.

Chiggers: Infestation with the larvae of the harvest mite, a small insect.

Chlamydia: A genus of small microorganisms that can produce cough, pneumonia, and inflammation of the eye in young children.

Chloramphenicol: An antibiotic that is used intravenously or orally to treat serious bacterial infections in children.

Cholera: A diarrheal illness caused by the bacterium *Vibrio cholerae.*

Cholesteatoma: A growth in the middle ear composed of old skin and debris. Can occur with chronic ear infections.

Chorea: Sudden, jerky movements of the arms, legs, and trunk. Often associated with rheumatic fever.

Chorioretinitis: Infection or inflammation of the chorion and retina, which are inner membranes of the eye.

Colorado Tick Fever: A tick-borne arboviral disease that causes fever, headache, fatigue, and a low white blood cell count.

Common Cold: An illness characterized by cough, fever, runny nose, and fatigue. Can be caused by many different viruses.

Congenital Infection: An infection that occurs before birth.

Conjunctivitis: Infection or inflammation of the conjunctivae, the membranes that line the eyelid and cover the outer portion of the eye.

Contagious: Able to be transmitted from one person to another.

Coxsackievirus: A member of the enterovirus group. Can produce infections in many organs, including the heart, gastrointestinal tract, and nervous system.

Croup: A viral illness of the upper airway. Most affected children have a characteristic barking, seal-like cough.

Cryptosporidiosis: A diarrheal illness due to infection with the protozoan *Cryptosporidium*.

CSF: Cerebrospinal fluid, the fluid that surrounds the brain and spinal cord.

CT: Computed tomography; also called CAT scan. A radiograph used to evaluate various areas of the body.

Cystitis: Infection or inflammation of the bladder.

Cytomegalovirus (CMV): A member of the herpesvirus group of viruses. Commonly shed by toddlers in group day care. When CMV infects a susceptible pregnant woman, the virus can be passed to the fetus, causing congenital infection.

D

Dermatitis: Infection or inflammation of the skin.

Dermatomyositis: An inflammatory condition that affects skin and muscles.

Dermatophytes: Fungi that infect the skin.

Diarrhea: Frequent loose or watery stools.

Diazepam (Valium®): A medication used as a muscle relaxant and as an anticonvulsant.

Diphtheria: An infectious disease caused by the bacterium *Corynebacterium diphtheriae*. Common symptoms are fever, sore throat, hoarse voice, and difficulty swallowing. Can be prevented by the DTP immunization.

Discitis: An inflammation or infection of the cartilage (disc) that lies between the bones of the spine.

Down Syndrome: Also known as trisomy 21 or mongolism. This is the most common chromosomal disorder.

Drug Fever: Fever produced as a side effect of drug therapy.

Dysentery: Bacillary dysentery is caused by bacteria and characterized by severe vomiting, water diarrhea, and abdominal cramping. Amebic dysentery is caused by an ameba and has similar symptoms.

E

Echovirus: A virus of the enterovirus group. Illnesses caused by this virus include meningitis, bronchitis, croup, the common cold, pneumonia, gastroenteritis, hepatitis, and infections of newborn infants.

Edema: Swelling of tissues due to increased water content of cells.

Ehrlichiosis: A disease caused by a tic-borne microorganism (*Ehrlichia* species). Infection is associated with fever, headache, muscle aches, and nausea or vomiting.

Empyema: A collection of pus within a body cavity.

Encephalitis: Infection or inflammation of brain tissue. Usually caused by a virus.

Endemic: Diseases that are regularly present in a geographic region.

Endocarditis: Infection of the lining of the heart. Usually caused by bacteria.

Endotoxin: A substance produced by bacteria. Has toxic effects, such as shock.

Enteritis: Infection or inflammation of the intestines.

Enterobius vermicularis: The cause of pinworms.

Enteroviruses: A group of viruses that includes echo, coxsackie, and polio viruses.

Epidemic: An outbreak of similar diseases or illnesses occurring at a particular time and place.

Epiglottitis: A serious infection or inflammation of the epiglottis, the structure that covers the entrance to the windpipe. Usually caused by the bacterium *Hemophilus influenzae* type b.

Escherichia coli: A bacterium (part of the body's normal flora) that causes many different childhood infections, including meningitis in infants and urinary tract infections.

F

Fasciitis: Infection of fascia, a connective tissue layer.

Fever: A temperature that exceeds the normal body temperature, usually 98.6°F (37°C) orally. (Rectal temperatures normally run a degree or so higher.)

Fifth Disease (Erythema infectiosum): A disease of young children characterized by rash of the face ("slapped cheek" appearance) and extremities. Caused by human parvovirus B19.

Flu: Influenza. A viral infection that can have respiratory and occasionally gastrointestinal symptoms.
Folliculitis: Infection of hair follicles.
Fomite: Inanimate object that participates in the transmission of infectious diseases.
Fungus: A mold. Many different fungi produce illness in humans.
Furunculosis: A pustular infection of the skin. Usually caused by the bacterium *Staphylococcus aureus*.

G

Gangrene: A destructive infection of skin, muscle, and other soft tissues. Associated with anaerobic bacteria.
Gastroenteritis: Infection of the stomach and intestines. Can be caused by viruses or bacteria.
Gentamicin: An antibiotic of the aminoglycoside group. Used to treat infections with Gram-negative bacteria, such as *E coli*.
Giardiasis: An illness with vomiting and diarrhea caused by the parasite *Giardia lamblia*. Epidemics can occur in day care and other settings where large numbers of children congregate.
Gingivostomatitis: An infection of the mouth, usually caused by herpes simplex virus type 1.
Glomerulonephritis: Infection or inflammation of the ducts of the kidney.
Gonorrhea: A sexually transmitted disease caused by the gonococcus *Neisseria gonorrhoeae*.
Gram Negative (or Gram Positive): A classification of bacteria based on the color reaction of the bacterial coat to a specific stain.
Granulocyte: Also known as a neutrophil. A white blood cell that can ingest and kill microorganisms, particularly bacteria.
Group A Streptococcus: The bacterium that causes strep throat, rheumatic fever, and scarlet fever.
Group B Streptococcus: A member of the streptococcus bacteria family. Causes serious infections in the newborn.
Guillain-Barré Syndrome: A postinfectious disorder that affects nerves after they exit the spinal cord. This disorder damages the myelin, which insulates the nerves.

H

Hand Foot and Mouth Disease: A viral illness with vesicular rashes on the hands, feet, and mouth. Usually caused by the coxsackieviruses.

Hemolytic-Uremic Syndrome: A postinfectious disorder of children; associated with acute anemia, low blood platelet count, and kidney failure.

***Hemophilus influenzae* Type b:** A bacterium that produces many different illnesses in children, including otitis media, pneumonia, meningitis, septic arthritis, and sinusitis. Invasive disease (eg, meningitis) can be prevented by vaccination.

Hepatitis: Infection or inflammation of the liver. Can be caused by bacteria, viruses, fungi, and certain commonly used medications.

Hepatitis A Virus: One cause of infectious hepatitis, usually spread by the fecal-oral route.

Hepatitis B Virus: The virus that causes serum hepatitis. Can be spread by blood transfusion, contact with saliva, or sexual contact.

Hepatitis C Virus: One virus that causes infectious hepatitis, usually spread by blood transfusion.

Herpangina: An illness with fever and lesions (ulcers or vesicles) of the throat and tonsils. Usually caused by enteroviruses.

Herpes Simplex Virus: A virus that can cause cold sores, genital lesions, encephalitis, and severe infections of young infants. Type 1 is usually associated with cold sores, type 2 with genital lesions.

Histoplasmosis: An illness caused by the fungus *Histoplasma capsulatum*. Usually affects the skin or lungs.

HIV-1: Human immunodeficiency virus type 1, the virus that causes AIDS.

Hookworm: Intestinal infection with the worms *Necator americanus* or *Ancylostoma duodenale*.

Hordeolum (Stye): An infection along the margin of the eyelid.

Human Herpesvirus Type 6: The virus that causes roseola.

Human Parvovirus B19: The virus that causes fifth disease (erythema infectiosum).

Hydrocephalus: Enlargement of the cerebrospinal fluid-filled spaces within and around the brain.

Hygiene: Practices that reduce transmission of viruses, bacteria, and parasites. Especially important are hand washing and prompt disposal of items such as diapers that may be contaminated with microorganisms.

I

Ileitis: Infection or inflammation of the last portion of the small intestine.

Immune Globulin: A concentrated form of γ globulin, or human antibodies, that can be given to prevent or modify infections (eg, hepatitis) in exposed individuals.

Immunity: The process by which the body develops mechanisms (eg, antibodies) to prevent or decrease the severity of an infection.

Immunization: A process in which the patient is given killed or innocuous microorganisms so that the body can develop immunity.

Immunodeficiency: The inability of the body to develop immunity. Can be the result of congenital or acquired processes.

Immunoglobulin (Ig): An antibody. The human body has five classes or types of immunoglobulins: IgA, IgM, IgG, IgE, and IgD.

Impetigo: A bacterial skin infection. Typically begins as a red spot and then progresses to a blister. Usually involves the face and hands.

Incidence: The number of persons affected by an illness or disorder during a given period of time.

Incubation Period: The time between exposure to a microorganism and the onset of illness.

Infantile Paralysis: Polio. The disease commonly associated with polio virus infection. Can be prevented by vaccination.

Infection: Invasion of a body tissue or fluid by a microorganism, such as a virus, bacterium, parasite, or fungus.

Infectious Mononucleosis: Also known as mono. An illness characterized by fever, fatigue, and swelling of lymph nodes. Can be caused by the Epstein-Barr virus or, less commonly, cytomegalovirus and other microorganisms.

Inflammation: A tissue reaction to injury or infection. Typical signs are swelling, redness, warmth, and pain.

Influenza: An illness, respiratory or gastrointestinal, caused by an influenza virus.

Interferon: A chemical produced by human cells. Inhibits the growth of viruses.

Isoniazid: An antibiotic used to treat tuberculosis.

J

Jaundice: Yellow appearance of skin or sclera (the white portion of the eye). Caused by elevation of the blood bilirubin level. One of the signs of hepatitis.

Jones Criteria: The signs of rheumatic fever (chorea, arthritis, heart murmur, skin rash, and skin nodules).

K

Kanamycin: An antibiotic of the aminoglycoside group. Similar to gentamicin.

Kawasaki Disease: A disease of young children. Typical symptoms include prolonged fever, peeling of the skin, sores of the tongue and mouth, inflammation of the eyes, and swelling of the joints.

Keratitis: Infection or inflammation of the cornea of the eye.

L

Labyrinthitis: Inflammation of the inner ear.

Legionnaires' Disease: A bacterial illness that usually affects the lung, brain, and gastrointestinal tract. Can be effectively treated by the antibiotic erythromycin.

Leprosy: A chronic bacterial infection of the skin or peripheral nerves.

Leptospirosis: An illness, usually with vomiting or diarrhea, caused by the bacteria of the *Leptospira* genus.

Leukocyte: A white blood cell.

Listeria monocytogenes: A bacterium that can cause serious illness (eg, meningitis) in infants or children with abnormal immune systems.

Lyme Disease: A tick-borne illness caused by the spirochete *Borrelia burgdorferi* that affects the skin, joints, and nervous system. Named for Lyme, Connecticut, the location of the first reported cases.

Lymphocyte: A type of white blood cell important in the body's defenses against viral infections.

M

Malaria: A chronic or relapsing illness with chills and fever. Caused by protozoa that are transmitted by mosquitos.

Mastoiditis: Infection of the mastoid air cells behind the ear.

Measles: A common childhood viral infection. There are two types: rubeola (hard measles) and rubella (3-day or German measles). Both types can be prevented by vaccination.

Meningitis: Infection of the covering (leptomeninges) of the brain and spinal cord.

Meningococcus: *Neisseria meningitidis,* a bacterium that causes meningitis and infection of the blood stream (sepsis).

Methicillin: An antibiotic of the penicillin group. Used to treat staphylococcal infections.

Metronidazole: An antibiotic used to treat infections caused by certain parasites and anaerobic bacteria.

Microcephaly: A head circumference that is markedly smaller than expected for a particular age.

Microorganism: A general name for microscopic organisms—viruses, bacteria, fungi, and parasites—that infect the human body.

Molluscum contagiosum: A viral infection of the skin. Similar to warts.

Monocyte: A white blood cell important in the body's defenses against infection.

Mucormycosis: A serious fungal disease. Often affects patients with diabetes mellitus.

Mumps: A common childhood illness. Characterized by fever, fatigue, and swelling of the parotid gland, a large salivary gland above the angle of the jaw.

Mycobacteria: A group of bacteria that includes *Mycobacterium tuberculosis*, the cause of tuberculosis. Other mycobacteria can produce infections of the lymph glands.

Mycoplasma pneumoniae: A microorganism that causes walking pneumonia and coldlike illnesses.

Myelitis: Infection or inflammation of the spinal cord.

Myocarditis: Infection or inflammation of cardiac muscle.

Myositis: Infection or inflammation of skeletal muscle.

Myringitis: Inflammation of the ear drum.

Myringotomy: A minor surgical procedure in which the ear drum is opened to allow fluid or pus to escape.

N

Nafcillin: An antibiotic of the penicillin family. Used to treat staphylococcal infections.

Necator americanus: The hookworm, a parasite that can infest the stomach and intestines.

Neisseria gonorrhoeae: The bacterium that causes gonorrhea, a sexually transmitted disease. This bacterium can also infect the eye of the newborn.

Neisseria meningitidis: The bacterium that causes meningococcal infections of the nervous system (meningitis) or blood stream (meningococcemia).

Neonate: An infant who is younger than 1 month.
Nephritis: Infection or inflammation of the kidney.
Neuritis: Inflammation of a nerve.
Neutrophil: A white blood cell important in the body's defenses against infection, especially with bacteria. Also called a granulocyte because it contains granules.
Nitrofurantoin: An antibiotic used to treat urinary tract infections.
Nocardia: Bacteria that can invade the liver, lung, or brain, especially in patients with abnormal immunity.
Norwalk Agent: A virus that produces a diarrheal illness, most commonly in adults.

O

Oophoritis: Also called ovaritis. Inflammation of the ovary.
Ophthalmitis: Infection or inflammation of the eye.
Orchitis: Infection or inflammation of the testes.
Organism: A living plant or animal.
Osteomyelitis: Infection of bone.
Otitis Media: Infection of the middle ear.

P

Pancreatitis: Infection or inflammation of the pancreas, an organ that produces insulin and digestive enzymes.
Parasite: An organism that lives on or in the body, deriving sustenance from the host.
Pasteurella Multocida: A bacterium transmitted to humans by dog or cat bites or scratches. Usually associated with a localized skin infection.
Pediculosis Capitis: Infestation with head lice.
Penicillin: A synthetic antibiotic (originally derived from a mold). The parent compound of many commonly used antibiotics (eg, ampicillin and amoxicillin).
Pericarditis: Infection or inflammation of the pericardium, the outer lining of the heart.
Pertussis: Also known as whooping cough. A bacterial infection that can produce episodes of severe coughing in young infants. Is fatal in some cases. Preventable by the DTP immunization.
Pharyngitis: Infection of the throat.
Pinworms: A common intestinal infestation with the worm *Enterobius vermicularis*. Itching around the anus is the most common symptom.

Plague: An illness characterized by fever, painful lymph node swelling, and occasionally pneumonia, caused by the bacterium *Yersinia pestis*.
Pleural Effusion: A collection of fluid within membranes surrounding the lung.
Pneumocystis carinii: A protozoan that causes pneumonia in infants and children with abnormal immune systems (eg, infants with acquired immunodeficiency syndrome, children receiving chemotherapy for malignancies, and infants with congenital abnormalities of the immune system).
Pneumonia: Infection of the lung.
Poliomyelitis (Infantile Paralysis): Infection of the spinal cord caused by the poliovirus. Preventable by vaccination.
Polyarteritis: Inflammation of blood vessels.
Polymyositis: Infection or inflammation of many muscles.
Prevalence: The number of persons affected by an illness or disorder at any one point in time.
Prophylaxis: A preventive measure. An example is the drug rifampin, which can be used to prevent *Hemophilus influenzae* infection.
Prostatitis: Infection or inflammation of the prostate gland.
Proteus mirabilis: A bacterial species that can cause urinary tract infections.
Protozoan: A single-celled organism (eg, *Pneumocystis carinii*).
Pseudomonas aeruginosa: A bacterium that can cause urinary tract infections in normal children and overwhelming infections in children with abnormal immune systems.
Pyelonephritis: Infection of the kidneys.

Q

Quinine: A medication used to treat malaria.
Quinsy: An abscess (a collection of pus and bacteria) that is adjacent to the tonsil.

R

Rabies: An uncommon encephalitic (affecting brain tissue) illness caused by the rabies virus and transmitted by the bites of infected animals.
Respiratory Syncytial Virus (RSV): A virus that causes coldlike symptoms in young infants and children.

Reye Syndrome: An illness that affects the liver and brain. Can follow many different childhood viral infections, including chickenpox and influenza.

Rheumatic Fever: A disorder associated with infection with group A streptococcal bacteria. Affects the heart, joints, skin, and nervous system.

Rhinoviruses: A group of viruses that can cause the common cold.

Rickettsia: Small microorganisms that share features of viruses and bacteria. Usually transmitted to humans by tick and flea bites.

Rifampin: An antibiotic used to treat certain fungal diseases and to prevent *Hemophilus influenzae* type b and *Neisseria meningitidis* infections in close contacts of infected individuals.

Ringworm: A fungal disorder that can affect the scalp (tinea capitis) or the body (tinea corporis).

Rocky Mountain Spotted Fever: An illness with rash, fever, and involvement of the brain. Caused by a rickettsial organism.

Roseola: an illness of young children characterized by fever (often quite high) and skin rash on the face, neck, and trunk. Caused by human herpesvirus type 6.

Rotavirus: A virus that causes diarrhea and, less often, vomiting in infants and young children.

Rubella: Also called 3-day measles. A mild viral infection. Can damage the fetus of a susceptible (nonimmunized) pregnant woman.

Rubeola: Also called hard measles. A viral infection characterized by high fever and rash.

S

St. Vitus' Dance: Also called chorea. A neurologic complication of rheumatic fever consisting of rapid, jerky movements of the arms, legs, and trunk.

Salmonella: A genus of bacteria that cause vomiting and diarrhea. *Salmonella typhi* causes typhoid fever.

Scabies: A skin infestation with the mite *Sarcoptes scabiei.*

Scarlet Fever: An illness with fever and a diffuse, red, blotchy skin rash caused by a group A streptococcus.

Sepsis: An illness with fever, and often shock. Caused by the presence of bacteria in the blood stream.

Serology: A blood test that measures antibodies to a specific microorganism. A person who lacks antibody is seronegative; a person who possesses antibody is seropositive.

Shigellosis: An illness with fever, vomiting, and diarrhea. Caused by shigella bacteria.

Shingles: A localized, pustular skin infection caused by the varicella-zoster virus, the same virus that causes chickenpox.

Sinusitis: Infection of the sinuses.

Smallpox: A viral illness characterized by fever and a poxlike rash of the face and extremities. Eliminated worldwide by immunization programs.

Spirochete: A group of spiral-shaped bacteria that cause several diseases, including syphilis and Lyme disease.

Spondylitis: Inflammation of the vertebral bodies of the spine.

Sporotrichosis: A fungal disease of the skin or subcutaneous tissues. Caused by *Sporotrichum schenckii*.

Staphylococci: A group of Gram-positive bacteria that cause many different infections in humans. Certain staphylococci normally reside on the skin.

Staphylococcus aureus: A bacterium that can cause infection of the lung, bones, joints, sinuses, and blood stream.

Stevens-Johnson Syndrome: A severe, sometimes fatal disorder involving skin and mucous membranes of the mouth and genitals. Has been associated with certain infections and medications.

STORCH: An acronym for a group of organisms that produce congenital infections (S = syphilis, T = toxoplasmosis, O = other infections, R = rubella, C = cytomegalovirus, H = herpes simplex). Also referred to as TORCH.

Streptococci: A group of Gram-positive bacteria that includes group A streptococci, the cause of strep throat.

Streptococcus pneumoniae: The pneumococcus, a bacterium that causes pneumonia, meningitis, and otitis media.

Streptomycin: An antibiotic.

Strongyloidiasis: A diarrheal illness caused by the worm *Strongyloides stercoralis*.

Subacute Sclerosing Panencephalitis (SSPE): A very rare neurologic disorder that can occur as a late complication of measles infection.

Sulfonamides: A group of antibiotics that have widespread applications.

Swimmer's Itch: Infestation of the skin by schistosomes (flatworms).

Sydenham's Chorea: Also known as St. Vitus' dance. A neurologic complication of rheumatic fever characterized by sudden, jerky movements of the body.

Synovitis: Inflammation of the joint space, most commonly of the hip.

Syphilis: A sexually transmitted disease caused by the spirochete *Treponema pallidum*.

T

Taenia saginata: The beef tapeworm.
Taenia solium: The pork tapeworm.
Tetanus: Also called lockjaw. A neurologic illness caused by infection with the bacterium *Clostridium tetani*. Effectively prevented by DTP immunization.
Tinea Capitis: Ringworm of the scalp.
Tinea Corporis: Ringworm of the body.
Tinea Pedis: Also called athlete's foot. A fungal infection.
T Lymphocytes: A group of white blood cells that provide immunity to viruses and other microorganisms.
Tonsillitis: Infection or inflammation of the tonsils.
TORCH: See STORCH.
Toxin: A chemical that has harmful effects on the body. Many bacteria produce toxins that can affect various organs.
Toxoplasmosis: An infection caused by the parasite *Toxoplasma gondii*.
Tracheitis: Inflammation or infection of the windpipe (trachea).
Tracheobronchitis: Infection or inflammation of the large air passages of the lungs.
Trachoma: Infection of the eye caused by *Chlamydia trachomatis*.
Treponema pallidum: The spirochete that causes syphilis.
Trichinosis: A systemic disease caused by the worm *Trichinella spiralis*. Usually acquired by eating raw or undercooked pork. Common symptoms are fever, muscle pain, weakness, nausea, and diarrhea.
Trichomoniasis: A genital infection caused by the protozoan *Trichomonas vaginalis*.
Tuberculosis: An illness caused by the bacterium *Mycobacterium tuberculosis*. Usually affects the lungs.
Tularemia: An illness with fever, chills, headache, and vomiting. Caused by the bacterium *Francisella tularensis*. Transmitted to humans from wild animals, ticks, and fleas.
Tympanocentesis: A procedure in which a needle is inserted through the ear drum to sample the contents of the middle ear.
Typhoid Fever: An illness with fever, fatigue, weight loss, rash, pneumonia, and neurologic symptoms. Caused by the bacterium *Salmonella typhi*.
Typhus: An illness with fever, headache, and rash. Caused by rickettsial organisms, which are transmitted to humans from ticks and lice.

U

Universal Precautions: A set of guidelines designed to prevent transmission of blood-borne microorganisms, especially HIV-1, the cause of AIDS. Includes the use of gloves, gowns, and eye protection in situations in which contamination by human blood or other body fluids is possible.

Ureaplasma: A genus of microorganisms closely related to the mycoplasmas. Can cause pneumonia in young infants.

Uremia: The presence of urine waste products in the blood stream. Associated with kidney failure.

Urethritis: Infection or inflammation of the urethra, a duct that carries urine from the bladder to the exterior of the body.

Urticaria: Hives.

Uveitis: Inflammation of the iris, ciliary body, and choroid of the eye.

V

Vaccine: A substance administered to prevent or decrease the severity of a disease.

Vaginitis: Infection or inflammation of the vagina.

Varicella-Zoster Virus: A member of the herpesvirus family. Causes chickenpox and shingles.

Variola: The smallpox virus.

Vasculitis: Inflammation of blood vessels.

Vesicle: A blisterlike skin rash.

Vibrio cholerae: The bacterium that causes cholera, an illness with vomiting and watery diarrhea.

Virulence: The intrinsic capacity of an organism to cause disease.

Virus: A small microorganism that cannot be seen with a light microscope.

Visceral Larva Migrans: An illness caused by the dog roundworm (*toxocara canis*) or cat roundworm (*Toxocara cati*). Signs include fever, enlargement of the spleen, involvement of the eye, and an alteration in the normal distribution of the types of white blood cells (eosinophilia).

Vulvovaginitis: Inflammation of the outer genital tract and vagina.

W

Wart: A small skin tumor caused by a member of the papovavirus group.

Waterhouse-Friderichsen Syndrome: A severe complication of meningococcal infection, characterized by shock, coma, skin rash, and abnormalities of the blood clotting mechanisms.

Whipworm: Infestation with the worm *Trichuris trichiura*. Symptoms include diarrhea and failure to thrive.

Whitlow: An infection of the fingertip. Usually caused by the herpes simplex virus.

Whooping Cough: Also called pertussis. An illness with severe, recurrent cough and fever. Caused by the bacterium *Bordetella pertussis*. Usually affects young infants.

X, Y, Z

Yersinia enterocolitica: A bacterium that can cause vomiting and diarrhea.

Zoster: Also called shingles. A skin infection caused by the varicella-zoster (chickenpox, shingles) virus.

Index

E

I

K

L

M

R

S

T